Memory Activity Book

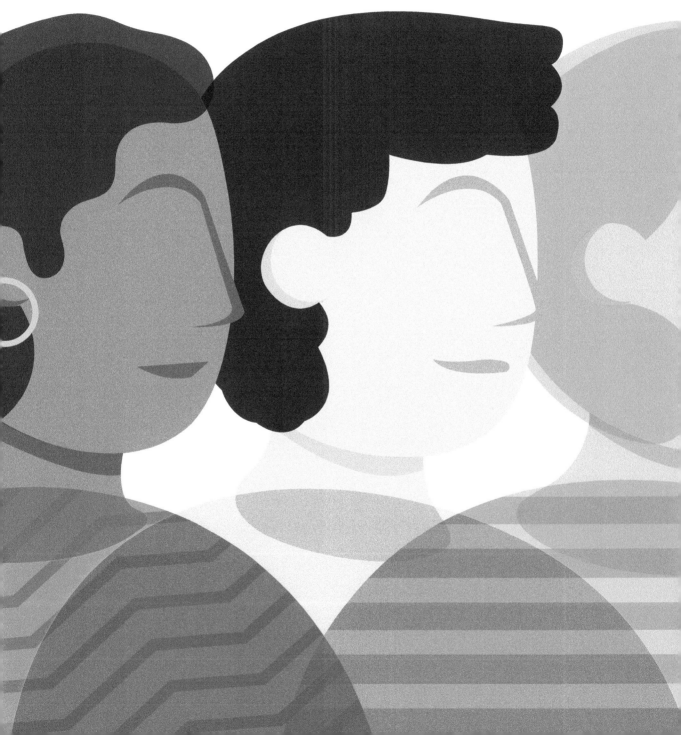

MEMORY
ACTIVITY BOOK

100+ BRAIN EXERCISES
TO SUPERCHARGE YOUR MEMORY

ALEXIS OLSON, PhD

ROCKRIDGE
PRESS

CONTENTS

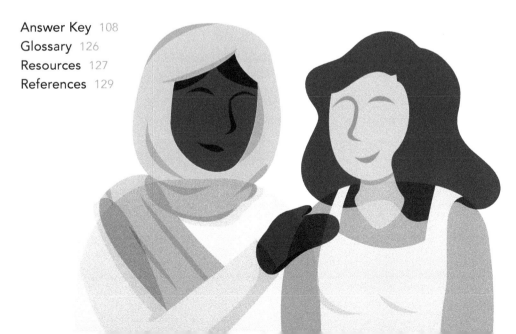

INTRODUCTION

In many ways, thinking is an art. We use our powers of organization and planning to direct information across the canvas of our minds. The speed at which we think builds energy, moving that information more quickly or slowly across the canvas. We create different effects in our mind, and we see the outcomes of our actions. We can be (somewhat) objective about our own thinking, allowing us to act as a director of thoughts or as an observer who frames certain thoughts in the foreground and moves others to the background.

As with art, some ways of thinking are more mainstream, whereas others are less common or understood. Over the years, I've seen many different arrangements of thinking abilities. As a neuropsychologist, I've aimed to understand these various arrangements and their inherent strengths and weaknesses. Of course, we all might yearn for the brain of Bradley Cooper's character in *Limitless*, who has unleashed all the magic of the mind and who is capable of seemingly infinite learning, recall, and problem solving. While an experience quite like that is unlikely to happen (at least in my lifetime), we *can* understand our own thinking abilities to a greater degree, leverage our strengths, and support our weaknesses through the artifices in our mind and environment.

Much of my focus is on the assessment of these abilities, often through quantifying the ability to think abstractly with language or space. Research and practice in this area reveal that patterns exist in how people perform in the different domains of thinking (e.g., attention and memory). We can also see how stress, nutrition, or other changes in the physical brain affect our ability to think. In my work in cognitive rehabilitation, I often review thinking strategies with people so they can maintain or enhance their level of functioning. Frequently, a relatively simple strategy, such as outlining a project beforehand or breaking large amounts of information into smaller pieces, can yield significant gains in everyday life. Although the strategies within this book have not been directly researched as a whole, they draw on aspects of such evidence-based practices as cognitive rehabilitation frameworks and research on the brain and thinking abilities.

In the field of psychology and brain science, the general consensus is that using our mind in novel and fun ways is one aspect of keeping it ready and able to optimally experience life. "Fun" is key, so we both engage in and enjoy the process of learning. The balance between challenging and stressing our mind is apparent in the findings of Dr. Mihaly Csikszentmihalyi (pronounced *cheek-sent-me-high*), who wrote about the flow state—that beautiful place where we feel fully engaged and joyfully challenged by our activity—in his book *Flow: The Psychology of Optimal Experience.* Novelty is also worth highlighting because if we keep doing the same thing day in and day out, we're unlikely to challenge our mind enough to access the full extent of our abilities. This book of activities is designed to give some food for thought and strategies on how to think and memorize effectively.

HOW TO USE THIS BOOK

While unavoidably interconnected, each chapter aims to represent a different type of thinking ability. Because of interdependency between thinking skills, you are welcome to jump to any chapter or progressively work your way through the book without missing a building block. Each chapter will begin with a description of that thinking skill, an explanation of how it is often used in everyday life, and suggestions for working more effectively with that particular ability. In each chapter, games progress in difficulty with increasing complexity, demand in pace, or delays in recall. To ensure you squeeze every ounce of usefulness out of this book, here are several tips for you to put into action:

1. **Designate a daily time** that you plan to dig into the activities or reflect on ways to apply them to your everyday life. Set an alarm or tie the act of reading this book to a routine activity, such as drinking your morning coffee or winding down from a daily walk.

2. **Commit to practicing** these exercises for at least 10 minutes per day. You can set a timer, if you'd like. Regular practice of a skill is what allows it to take root. Find a time frame that works for you; start small and add a couple of minutes each time, as you go. Many of these activities can be repeated in novel ways, so practicing can go on and on.

3. **Team up** and work through the activities with a friend. We're social animals. Science shows we thrive on friendly (and even sometimes unfriendly) competition. It pushes us to stay focused and go that extra mile. When left to our own devices, we might simply throw in the towel.

4. **Set a goal and revise as necessary** to keep yourself motivated and to achieve a sense of accomplishment. Whether a friend is joining you or not, remain competitive with yourself. See if you can repeat certain activities with alternative categories and do even better the next time.

5. **Imagine that you'll be teaching** someone else about this skill (or actually do teach it). We tend to remember things better when we have to describe our knowledge to others.

6. **Start where you can** and progressively build up to harder activities. If you find you're getting hung up on any one game and becoming frustrated, take a break and a breath. Phone a friend (needing a trivia answer is a great reason to reach out to those we love).

7. **Be compassionate with yourself.** We're often great at criticizing ourselves, even if that does nothing more than put our spirits in the dumps and distract us from what we want to do. As is often said in various forms in therapy, "You are where you are." Once we truly accept our strengths *and* weaknesses, we can better utilize energy otherwise spent fighting with our critical self.

8. **Apply the strategy** to some aspect of your daily life after working through an activity. Some of the chapter introductions offer insights and suggestions on how to do this, but feel free to think outside the box. In what ways might you use a new strategy at home, in your office, or with friends? I'm sure you'll come up with at least a few ways to put them to good use.

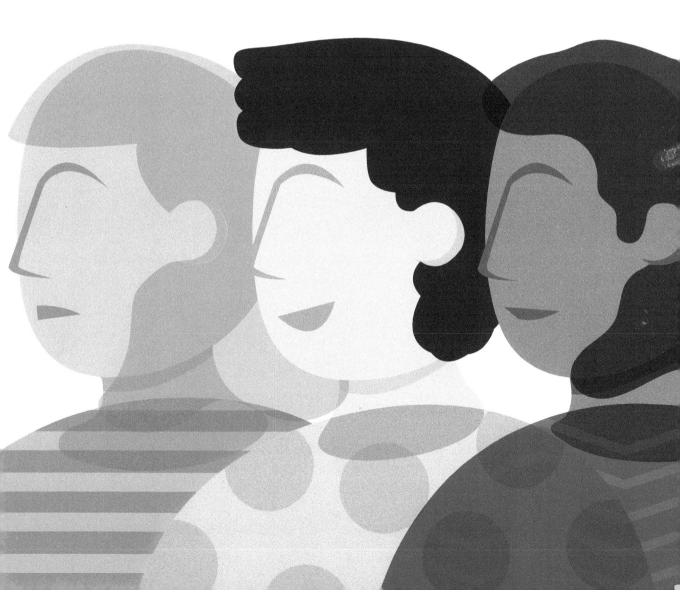

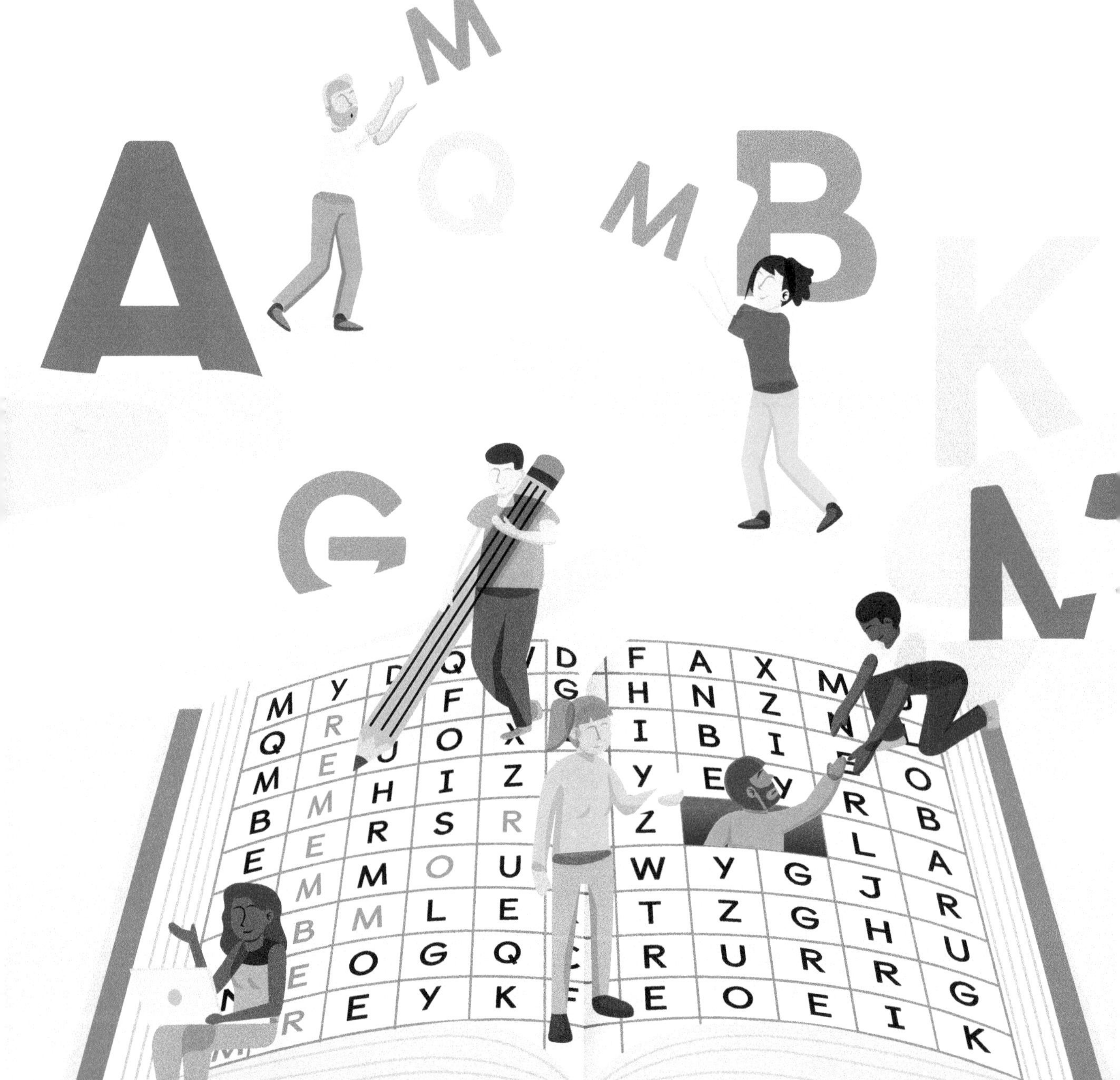

CHAPTER 1

WHAT IS MEMORY, AGAIN?

If you tell the truth, you don't have to remember anything.
—Mark Twain

Mark Twain undervalued the importance of memory in his rationale for telling the truth. If it weren't for memory, we'd be both unable to plan effectively for the future, as well as blissfully unaware of any past mistakes. We can rely on others to fill in some blanks, but for most of us, carrying our own recollection of events is important. It allows us to form a life narrative, give weight to certain moments over others, and merge our realities with other people's perspectives as we mutually recall those details that populate our lives. We make use of various types of memory, as well as supportive thinking skills, in our daily life.

Our memories of this moment, our ability to hold all the details in mind, such as the words in this sentence, depend on a type of memory called working memory. It functions somewhat like a drawing board with ink lasting a matter of seconds if not sketched over again. The bigger the drawing board, the more information you can work with. Yet, as science has shown us, each of our drawing boards are roughly the same—with about seven (some say four) slots for bits of information. But what if there existed ways to optimize this workable space, ways to be more efficient? Indeed, there are such ways, which we will cover in this book. We will also discuss the other players in memory formation, which include cognitive abilities such as attention and organization, and we'll even touch on contributions from emotions and daily behaviors, such as sleep and good nutrition.

The bulk of this book will focus on cognitive strategies that facilitate the ability to absorb information, place it meaningfully in your mind, and effectively locate and extract it when needed. To optimize this precious ability, we'll review ways of organizing information more efficiently (similar to a game of Tetris). Organization is considered an executive functioning (EF) skill. When you think of EF skills, think of a corporate executive and what their job involves: planning, prioritizing, monitoring progress, adapting to changes, and following through on a project. As you might have inferred, memory is key to each of these duties. You may also have picked up on a bit of a chicken-egg relationship here, since one thinking skill influences the quality of another thinking skill, which returns the influence. Because of this, improvement in one thinking skill, like organization, offers improvements in the other, like memory, and vice versa.

Some thinking skills, such as attention and processing speed, are more foundational. By this I mean they underlie and potentially limit or expand other abilities, such as memory or planning, with less (though still some) influence in return. These foundational abilities seem to function like a funnel. The longer you can sustain attention or the more quickly you gather information into your mind, generally the more efficiently you can execute a task, like finding a face in a crowd or balancing your checkbook. To some degree, we can train in various strategies to optimize performance in these areas.

MEMORY AND THE BRAIN

While all parts of the brain are important for various purposes, such as keeping your heart beating or moving your eyes across this page, certain parts of the brain play a key role in memory. Additionally, memory comes in different forms, each form drawing on different parts of the brain.

The famous hippocampus (you have one on either side of your brain) is named for its resemblance to the shape of a seahorse and is located toward the middle lower portion of your brain. The hippocampus is the keystone of memory. As seen in a famous neuroscience patient named H.M., when both hippocampi (plural for hippocampus) are removed, the ability to form most (but not all) long-term memories vanishes. The main type of memory associated with the hippocampus is declarative memory, meaning you can declare it to the world in some way, like talking or writing about it.

Procedural memory is a type of nondeclarative memory, meaning you may not be able to tell people what you know how to do, but you can show them. Memory for how to carry out an action like riding a bicycle (procedural memory) relies, in part, on the cerebellum (from Latin, meaning "little brain"). Even if your hippocampi were damaged, you could still learn many of the fun things in life using your cerebellum, like how to row a boat, play catch, or strum the guitar. Another structure, the basal ganglia, assists in this type of memory, as well as aspects of working memory. A basal ganglia structure exists on each side of the brain, and it looks a bit like a large, curled-up tadpole. Besides helping you learn motor tasks, these structures are also associated with operant conditioning, the type of learning that is driven by reward or punishment. Think about what happens when you remember to shower or to lock your car door; you get the reward of smelling and feeling nice with the former and avoid the punishment of someone stealing your belongings with the latter.

How does our brain determine what is worth remembering? Our emotional response, which is driven by our amygdala, plays a part in this process. Located just above each hippocampus, the amygdala is a little almond-shaped structure that facilitates learning of emotionally charged material, especially information related to situations eliciting fear. The general rule is that a stronger emotional response leads to better memory formation; however, too much or too little emotional charge can hamper memory formation. Generally, we're looking for a sweet spot of engaged but not overwhelmed. Our emotional processing of memories also occurs when we return to a memory. A little rewriting of the event happens on such recollection. In a sense, we leave our emotional fingerprints each time we revisit the memory, coloring it with the mood we are in when we recall it. This is part of the process that allows people to work through traumatic memories to feel safer and more at peace.

We've highlighted just a few of the key regions of the brain we rely on for our memories. The truth is that many parts of the brain work together to form each memory, retain it, and revisit it at a later time.

MYTH BUSTING

We've all heard a tall tale or two about the body, maybe even the brain specifically. Here are a handful of myths you should feel free to debunk the next time you hear them:

1. **We only use 10 percent of our brains.** This is a fun one because, if true, it would mean we have some amazing untapped potential. Alas, according to the Mayo Clinic, we're likely to use 100 percent of our brains over the course of a day. We do have different types of brain cells, some involved in active thinking and others known as support cells (e.g., glial cells are your brain's housekeeping cells, which work to tidy up the mess of old or damaged cells), but all are generally useful and used.

2. **At some age your brain stops growing.** While early life provides the bulk of brain growth, parts of our brain generate new cells throughout our entire life. In particular, these sites are the hippocampus (memory center) and olfactory bulb (your sense of smell). Even if your brain isn't making new cells, it continues to adapt through the process of neuroplasticity. This means pathways between neurons (brain cells) are constantly being altered in response to your interaction with the world, making active engagement so important.

3. **We remember things exactly as they happened.** You've probably heard of people whose minds are "like a steel trap." While some people's memories are better than others, our recollection is often colored by what was important to us at the time we formed the memory, as well as how we're feeling when we recall the memory. Mood congruence, as this is called, means that if you're happy, you're likely to recall the happy parts of a memory, and so on. It also explains in part why eyewitness testimony is notoriously unreliable, since witnesses are likely to be influenced by how questions are phrased, affecting which details they recall accurately.

4. **Memory loss is normal and unavoidable.** Some memories will take a little more time to access than others. However, being frequently forgetful of significant life details, like main points of recent conversations or familiar people, is a reason to visit with your doctor. In fact, our fund of information (known as crystallized intelligence) continues to grow as we age. Staying mentally active at any age can protect against declines in aspects of thinking, as well as delay the onset of dementia. A key to keeping memory sharp is practicing adaptive strategies, like using cues and ways of organizing information, such as those covered in this book.

5. **You can learn by listening while you sleep.** This myth is a shade more believable than "sleeping with a book under your pillow will let you learn its material." However, it's just as untrue. If you're truly sleeping, you might incorporate some imagery or items into your dreams from the material you hear, but the odds that you will use the information in any meaningful way are slim to none. Plus, you're more likely to disturb your sleep if you have audio playing throughout the night. It's best to learn the information the old-fashioned way, while awake.

6. **You can't learn a new language as an adult.** It's true that if you learn a language after your early teenage years, you're likely to always speak it with an accent. However, while some aspects of learning a

new language may be more laborious or take longer as we age, we're definitely capable of learning a new language. In fact, learning a new language is associated with greater creativity, flexibility, and fluency in one's native language. Immersion is the best way to learn a new language, as it commands your full attention and provides cues from all angles for better recall of new words and principles.

7. **People are either left-brained or right-brained.** As discussed earlier, specific areas of the brain serve certain functions. Some people are stronger in one skill than another, but scientists have found no evidence that left-brained or right-brained people exist. We rely on both halves of the brain for different components of thought and perform best when both sides communicate with each other to solve different aspects of a problem. So, whether you're artistic or mathematical, you're strengthening the networks on both sides of your brain generally to a similar degree.

MEMORY TRICKS

As you'll be practicing throughout this book, keep in mind the following tips and tricks on how to more easily retain information and recall it later:

1. **Teach it.** Practice explaining what you want to remember to a 12-year-old (i.e., keep it simple), particularly for complex or multipart concepts. Repeat your instruction until you feel like you've filled in any gaps and boiled it down to the necessary parts.

2. **Story method.** We humans love stories. We often think in narratives. So, to remember bits of unrelated information, simply make a story out of the pieces of information you wish to recall. For example, if you have a list of errands (e.g., feed the dog, get the mail, deposit checks at the bank, call Luis), you can make up the following story: "Luis found a dog in the bank's mailbox." Typically, only one cue is needed per item, and it can be one word (e.g., "Luis" means to call Luis) to make for a tidy little story.

3. **Number rhyming.** This is a basic but effective trick. Create a rhyme with the important numbers, such as a date. (Hint: You may not need to use all numbers in the rhyme.) This can work for dates, such as "Remember, remember the 5th of November." You're just rhyming the details with the date to be remembered. Other examples are "776 heavenly Olympic tricks" (to recall the year of the earliest Olympic games, 776 BCE) and "1348 a thirsty plague through England's gates" (to remember the 1348 arrival of the Black Death to England). Try it with a date you'd like to keep in mind.

4. **Analogies.** Tie new bits of information to some of your prior knowledge, especially those hobbies or interests you value highly. Let's say you're a baker and you're trying to remember historical figures. You can elaborate on each person based on their accomplishment or personality by aligning it with a baked good or an ingredient. For example, Amelia Earhart is like an angel food cake or baking powder because they are all associated with rising. This works particularly well if you're trying to remember names of new acquaintances (e.g., Fred the lemon tart because he has a sharp sense of humor).

5. **The body list.** This is similar to a technique called the method of loci (Latin for "method of place"), but instead of using your surroundings, you use your body parts. Start with the top of your head, then associate the items you want to remember with parts of your body. For a grocery list, imagine balancing oranges on the top of your head, pasting napkins to your forehead, covering your ears with cups, coating your eyes with jam, getting whipped cream on your nose, and putting cocoa on your lips. Now you have all the items on your list associated with body parts.

6. **Time lines.** This time you're using space to place points on a time line. Imagine a familiar space, preferably one that has clear midpoints and delineating lines. For example, if you're into soccer, you can use the field as a means of remembering time lines by placing them in

different positions on the field or before or after the dividing lines (e.g., midline, penalty box). You can use the dates themselves, such as spreading the last 50 years of political events across the chosen space, or less discrete events, such as what happened in the course of a road trip (which can be more about the *order of events* than the exact date/time something happened).

7. **Note cards for errorless learning.** Typically, you just need to remember your general points, so making a list of word cues using the story method might work. Other times you want to learn information word for word. In the latter case, you can break up the information, such as a speech, into paragraphs and then write each sentence of the first paragraph on its own note card. Repeat with each paragraph. Errorless learning means you correct yourself after each error, repeatedly practicing until there are no errors. Shuffle through the note cards and discard those you have memorized until you have only those left that you are mastering through more frequent exposure.

8. **Set it to music.** Beyond putting you in a good mood, the beat and lyrical space of songs can be used to remember details. Those of you who wrote a song about the quadratic equation in high school would know (I'm not the only one). You can keep the tune as simple as "Twinkle, Twinkle, Little Star" or as complex as your favorite Queen song. For the former tune, to remember elements of the periodic table, you could sing: "Hydrogen one and helium two, lithium beryllium end in um, too." You can make the song as information-packed or as true to the lyrics as works for you. Sing it through a few times, and it'll stick.

BRAIN BOOSTERS

In addition to the techniques and exercises you'll learn in this book, there are lots of other ways you can boost your brain power.

1. **Catch quality Zs.** Your brain needs at least six hours of sleep nightly to tidy itself up, including shifting memories into long-term storage and cleaning and repairing brain tissues. If you're having trouble, look into how to make a good bedtime routine (see Resources) and/or talk to your doctor.

2. **Good nosh.** Eating healthy foods will not only provide your mind with the nutrients it needs, but you'll also get long-lasting energy instead of a sugar crash. Fewer crashes ensures a more even mood and clearer thinking. Make room for sweet potatoes, lean proteins, whole grains, and leafy greens, such as broccoli, kale, and spinach. Snack on berries (packed with flavonoids) and walnuts (loaded with healthy fats).

3. **Supplements.** Check with your doctor to see if your body needs supplements for optimal function. People commonly need to supplement with vitamin B complex (especially when stressed) and vitamin D (especially in winter). Some herbs are touted for brain-boosting power, although the scientific jury is out on many of them.

4. **Exercise.** I can't say enough about the benefits of exercise. Move your body "vigorously" for 25 minutes per day, meaning you're likely sweating lightly and having only mild difficulty carrying on a conversation. Exercise also boosts mood and has been found in some studies to be as effective as medication in managing mood symptoms.

5. **Playtime.** Enjoy a game of cards, croquet, or Scattergories. Our brains love challenges, but they're often stressed by risk. When we play, we remove the risk while asking our brain to creatively face challenges. This boosts feel-good brain chemicals while limiting the effects of stress on the body and mind.

6. **Social time.** The "just right" amount of social time varies from person to person. Social time with others can provide us with a sense of security and relatedness that reduces stress and engages our faculties. It's worth making the trek to a neighbor's house, going on a hike with company, or ringing up an old friend.

7. **Quiet time.** After all that play and social time, our brains like to be balanced out with restorative quiet time. This might mean doing a meditative activity, like raking leaves or practicing breathing exercises—time when we can witness our mind as it wanders and returns, without demanding too much of it.

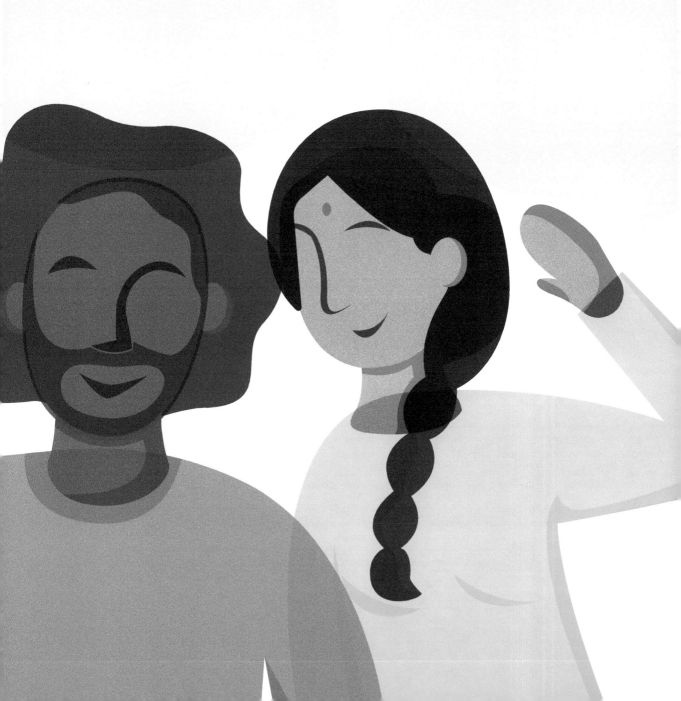

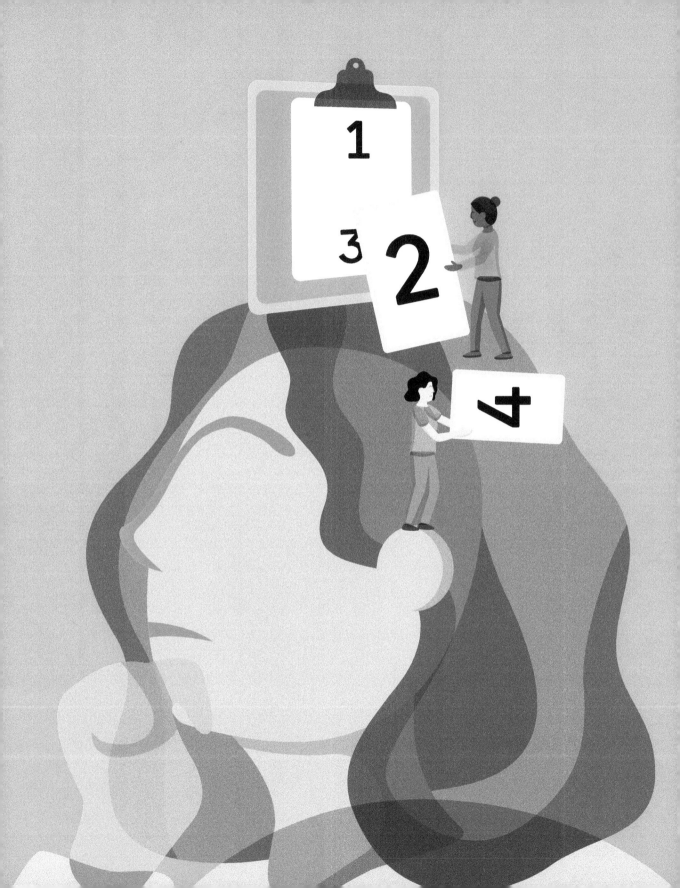

CHAPTER 2

REPEAT AFTER ME

(Short-Term Memory)

Hearing is one of the body's five senses.
But listening is an art.
—Frank Tyger, American cartoonist

Primary memory, also known as short-term memory, is composed of all of the sensations that arrive as impressions on your consciousness. It's a lot like a Buddha Board (aka Zen Board or Magic Paper) that you draw on with water, which then evaporates over a short period of time. If you don't retrace the same lines with water, the image disappears. Similarly, primary memory relies on and is refreshed or replaced by incoming sensory information. This makes primary memory a bit squirrelly. We're constantly exposed to new sensory information. If we're not able to harness the sensory information arriving in primary memory (using our working memory), we're likely to lose it. There is some debate about just how much information can be held in primary memory, but some say about four pieces of information can stay put in our minds at a time. You might be thinking, "Wait, I can remember more than four numbers someone tells me or four words on a page." You're right. But the way you recall more is by using strategies and other capacities, such as working memory, which we'll get into later in this book.

Attention is key to primary memory. It's like a spotlight: It can be *diffuse* or *focal*. Diffuse attention is broad, sweeping. It takes in the broad configuration of a scene and its details (e.g., where people are standing and what the weather looks like). Focal attention homes in on sensory information from a small area, such as staring into a tree and trying to make out whether a bird's eye is open or closed. Switching attention is another aspect of attention, but it looks different. It occurs, for instance, as you move your focus between tracking the path of a runner and observing the time on your stopwatch. Later in this book we'll work on switching your attention, but for now we'll focus on exercising broad attention to details and relationships among different sights and sounds and ways to track those details effectively.

In our everyday lives, we utilize primary memory frequently. While primary memory is rather limited, we can work with it using the technique of chunking (clumping information into sets) as well as using our visuospatial sketch pad. The visuospatial sketch pad is what it sounds like. It's the mental chalkboard your mind uses to retain and work with visual information such as shapes, colors, and patterns. Practicing using your visuospatial sketch pad to arrange objects in groups or in the configuration of a square can help you recall objects a short while later. You can also use this method to remember phone numbers by drawing patterns/shapes on the keypad. As we go through our day, we rely heavily on our senses and the information they provide, such as when monitoring the road while driving, engaging in conversations, or even listening to music.

See which of the above strategies you can use to solve the following activities.

CARD SORTING

Exercise 1

Using a deck of playing cards, make two five-card piles with the same card ranks (e.g., 1, 2, 3, jack, queen). Shuffle one five-card pile and lay the cards in a line faceup, from left to right. Study those cards for 10 to 20 seconds. Flip them all facedown. Then, using your memory, arrange the other pile of matching cards in the same order. Flip the facedown cards over to see how many match. Add more cards for additional difficulty.

> TIP: *Although relying only on visual input would make this more of a primary memory task, you can "chunk" any patterns of colors or numbers, using working memory to enhance later recall (e.g., dividing cards into chunks of 1-2-3 and jack-queen).*

Exercise 2

Using the same two piles (with the same card ranks, e.g., 1, 2, 3, jack, queen), shuffle each and lay all the cards from one pile faceup in the shape of a circle. Study those cards for 10 to 20 seconds. Flip them all facedown. Then, next to the first circle, arrange the other pile of matching cards in the same order. Flip them over to see how many match. If you're having trouble, decrease the number of cards until it's challenging but fun.

CONTINUED

CARD SORTING *Continued*

Exercise 3

Using playing cards, lay any nine cards in the shape of a plus sign (+)—five left to right, two above the middle card, and two below the middle card. Take a photo. Pick up and shuffle the placed cards, then try to lay them out in the same configuration as before. Check your accuracy using the photo of the original layout.

Exercise 4

Using playing cards, lay nine cards faceup in the shape of a square—a 3-by-3-card grid. Study the cards for about 30 seconds, then flip them facedown. Try to guess each card, one at a time. Verify your accuracy by flipping over the card; either leave it faceup or, for an extra challenge, flip it facedown before guessing your next card.

EYE-CATCHERS
Exercise 1

Study the following picture for 30 seconds. Turn to the next page and answer the following questions, taking your best guesses:

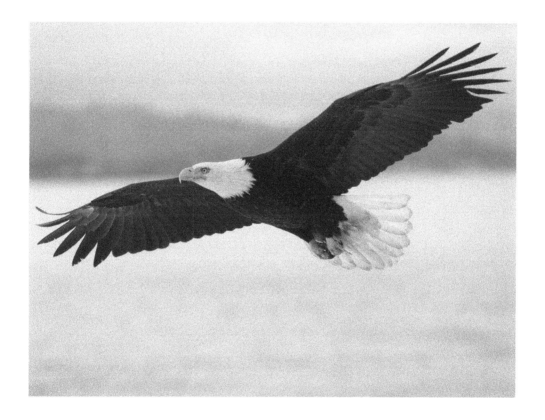

CONTINUED

Exercise 1 *Continued*

1. How many feather tips are at the end of each wing?

_____

2. Which direction is the eagle facing?

_____

3. Is the tail pointing up, down, to the side, or at an angle?

_____

4. What color is the eagle's head?

_____

5. Are the eagle's talons open or closed?

_____

Exercise 2

Study the following picture for 30 seconds. Turn to the next page and answer the following questions:

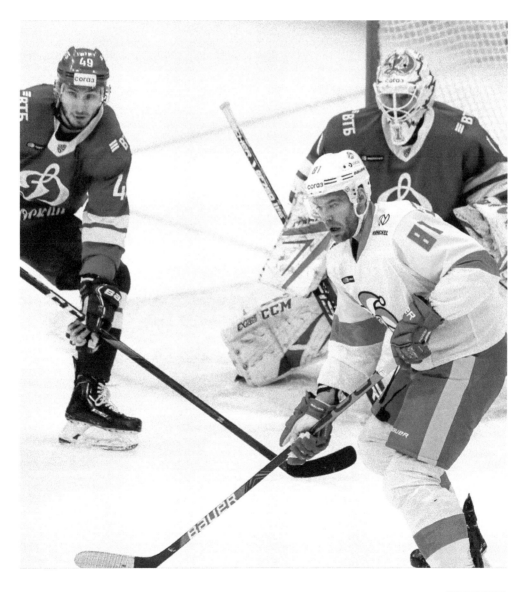

CONTINUED

Exercise 2 *Continued*

1. How many people are in the scene?

   _____

2. What colors are present?

   _____

3. Is there a hockey puck in the image?

   _____

4. Is there a face shield on any of the helmets?

   _____

5. What color is the goalie's jersey?

   _____

Exercise 3

Study the following picture for 30 seconds. Turn to the next page and answer the following questions:

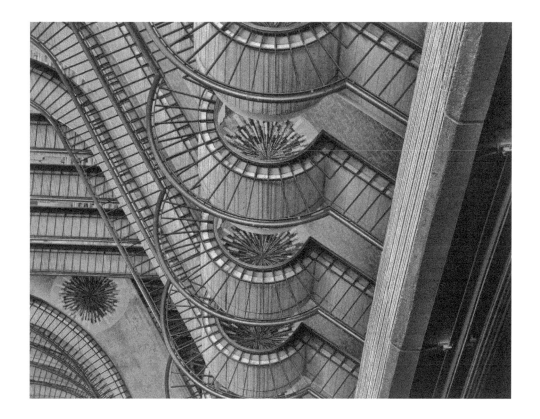

CONTINUED

Exercise 3 *Continued*

1. Is an elevator present?

    _____

2. What color(s) is the floor?

    _____

3. How many semicircular railings are visible?

    _____

4. Are there any people present?

    _____

Exercise 4

Study the following picture for 30 seconds. Turn to the next page and answer the following questions:

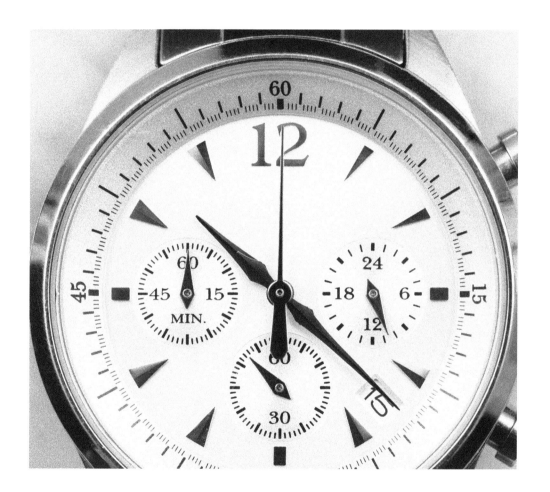

CONTINUED

Exercise 4 *Continued*

1. What numbers are on the outermost ring of the clockface?

_____

2. How many small inner dials are there?

_____

3. How many hands on the small inner dials are generally pointing up?

_____

4. What number is the second hand pointing to?

_____

5. How many hands are present, including both the watch face and inner dials?

_____

Exercise 5

Study the following picture for 30 seconds. Turn to the next page and answer the following questions:

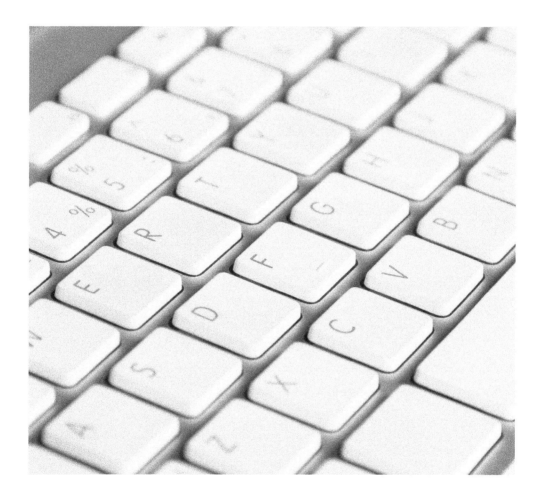

CONTINUED

Exercise 5 *Continued*

1. How many rows of keys are there?

_____

2. Name three letters that you can see.

_____

3. How many rows of letters are there for sure (that you can see letters on)?

_____

4. How many rows of numbers are there?

_____

5. How many numbers are visible (in focus or not)?

_____

TAKE IN THE VIEW

Exercise 1

With a pen and paper in hand (or the space on page 29), look at one side of a room in your house for 30 seconds. Look away and put pen to paper to draw or write as many details as are in your mind. See how proportional you can make your figures, such as furniture. Then look back and see how your recall compares to real life.

> TIP: *If drawing isn't your thing, consider using a piece of grid paper to gauge location and proportion better. Later switch to freestyle on a blank piece of paper.*

Exercise 2

Using a pen and paper (or the space on page 29), draw your own detailed design/scene. Study the design as closely as you can for one minute, then flip the paper over (or get a new piece of paper) and draw the design again. See how closely the designs match.

CONTINUED

Exercise 3

With a pen and paper in hand (or the space on page 29), look at a magazine cover for 30 seconds. Look away and put pen to paper to draw or write as many details as are in your mind. Try to place the words and images close to their original location. Then look back and see how your recall compares to the original.

Exercise 4

Pull up an online map of an unfamiliar city. Pick three or more destinations and generate directions. Study the line of travel. Then, on a sheet of white paper (or the space on page 29), see how accurately you can draw the line of travel. Check back with the map to see how correctly you've identified turns and gauged distances.

Draw here!

PALM READING
Exercise 1

Using the map of palm points, use your left index finger to draw on your right palm in the order of the following numbers (like connect the dots). Then flip to page 32 and choose which two shapes you drew on your hand from the designs listed for this activity:

1. **32451**

2. **35923**

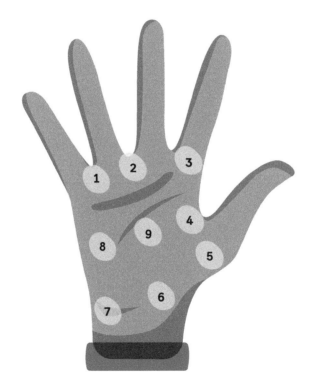

Exercise 2

Again, using the map of palm points, use your left index finger to draw on your right palm in the order of the following numbers (like connect the dots). Then flip to the next page and choose which two shapes you drew on your hand from the designs listed for this activity:

1. **294817**

2. **928427**

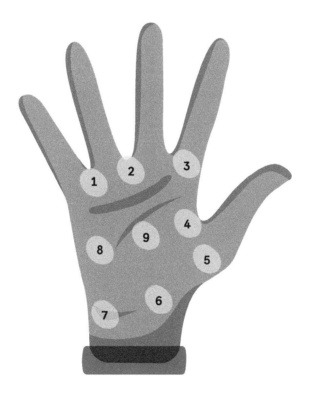

PALM READING

For Exercise 1

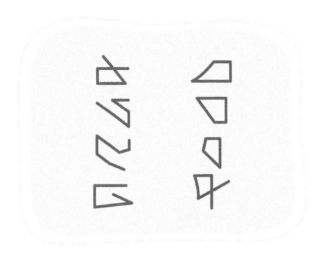

For Exercise 2

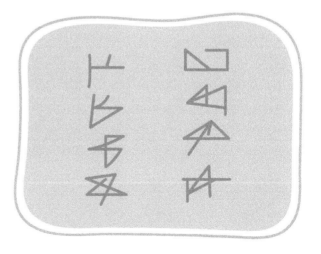

TUNING IN

Exercise 1

Turn on an unfamiliar song. Listen for 10 seconds, then hit pause. Hum as many notes as you can from memory. (Consider recording yourself as means of double-checking.) Hit rewind and see how many notes you've correctly hit.

Exercise 2

Turn on an unfamiliar movie or show. Listen for five seconds of dialogue, then hit pause. Say as many lines as you can from memory. (Consider recording yourself as means of double-checking.) Hit rewind and see how many words you've correctly remembered.

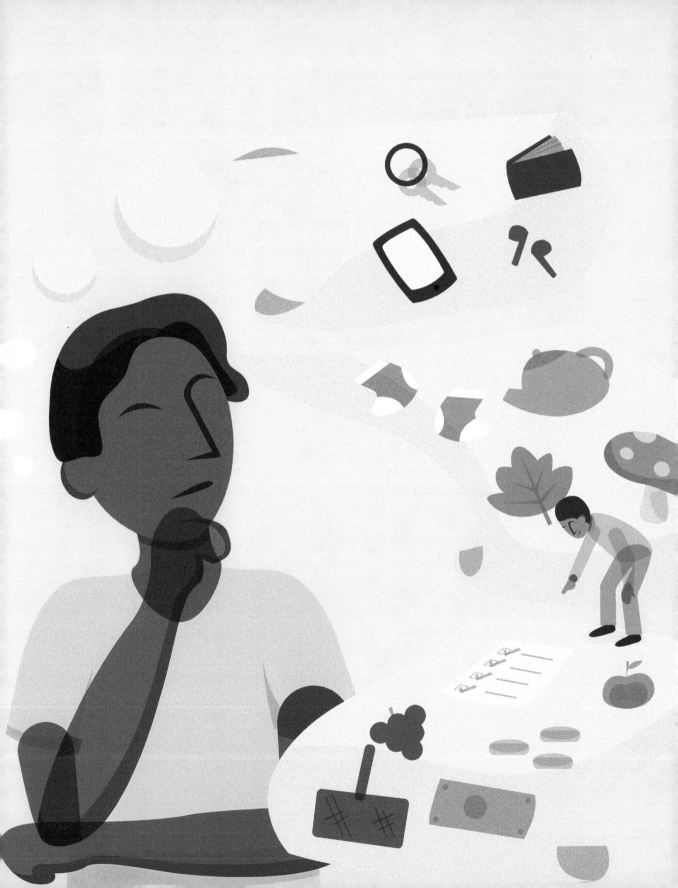

CHAPTER 3

WATCH IT WORK

(Working Memory)

*Working memory is the fundamental function
by which we break free from reflexive . . . reactions
to gain control over our own thoughts.*
—Earl K. Miller, Mikael Lundqvist, and André M. Bastos; MIT researchers

Without working memory, we'd be stuck doing whatever reflexes and conditioned behaviors we had developed. You wouldn't be able to calculate a tip in your head or tailor a verbal response before saying it. Life would be a lot simpler, though not as easy. Since we *are* able to use working memory, we can hold more than one thing in mind and organize information to best suit our purposes. Such purposes might include visualizing how puzzle pieces fit together or remembering the details of the coffee your friend wanted you to order—pretty fundamental stuff when it comes to day-to-day life. Working memory allows us not only to work with incoming information, like what someone is saying to us, but also to call up and manipulate previously learned information. You might liken working memory to a pan, where you put ingredients from the store (incoming sensory information) and the cupboard (long-term memory). The bigger the pan is, the more space there will be to work with your ingredients without them falling out. Working memory is often thought of as a subtype of short-term memory, specifically involving the manipulation of information.

Working memory is, in my opinion, one of the most "hackable" cognitive abilities we have. We can strategize our way to holding more and more information in mind. *Chunking*, or the practice of breaking up larger sets of information into smaller portions, is often done subconsciously, but sometimes we need to make an added effort to chunk information. For example, to learn the sequence "MLSFISFSD," I might chunk it into groups of three letters, making it easier to store ("MLS-FIS-FSD"). Many of these strategies rely somewhat on long-term memory, such as our familiarity with acronyms or number groups (e.g., 911800 breaks down to the emergency phone number 911 and the 800 toll-free number area code). However, a strategy can also be simply organizational, where information is organized into subsets of information that are related to each other in novel ways. For example, if you want to remember the name of each person at your job, school, or neighborhood, you could break them into groups by department, class, or household, respectively. Similarly, you can organize visual material into certain configurations or shapes to make it easier to recall (or to cue when you're forgetting a piece of the picture). See which of the above strategies (and those from chapter 1) you can use with the following activities.

CHUNKING

Exercise 1

Chunk the following objects into categories. Try to come up with a few different chunking options (e.g., office supplies, foods, animals):

BLUE JAY · RED ROBIN · CARROT · POTATO · DOVE · ELEPHANT · DOG · PAPER · PEN · PLANT · TANGERINE · ERASER · RASPBERRY

Exercise 2

Chunk the following states into categories. Try to come up with a few different chunking options:

NEVADA · FLORIDA · CALIFORNIA · NEBRASKA · MAINE · NORTH DAKOTA · MONTANA · TEXAS · VERMONT · CONNECTICUT

Exercise 3

Chunk the following objects into categories. Try to come up with a few different chunking options:

FRISBEE · SOCKS · PEN · FIREWOOD · CARDS · MATCHES · T-SHIRT · SKIS · GLOVE · BOOTS · GASOLINE · BASKETBALL

Exercise 4

Chunk the following people into categories. Try to come up with a few different chunking options:

BOB · JILL · FRANCINE · JEAN · FRANK · JIM · BRENDA · ADAM · BRITTANY · ABIGAIL

SPATIAL RELATIONS

Exercise 1

You're standing on a corner, holding a sign that points toward your garage sale to your left. You look across the street to your right and see a friendly dog facing you that is off leash. To the dog's right across the street is a girl with her back to you. On her left across the street is a car parked facing the girl.

1. Can the people in the car see your sign?

2. Can the girl clearly see the people in the car if she's looking straight ahead?

3. If the dog crossed the street to its right, toward the girl, could it then see your sign (and would it have to turn around its head)?

TIP: Chunk the instructions into steps. Create a mental map, maybe even using a familiar intersection. Use your body to gauge the positions of the various subjects in the exercise.

Exercise 2

Without using paper, solve the following word problem: You're heading south toward your favorite lake. A detour requires you to take two left turns, then five right turns, then a U-turn, and then one final left-hand turn.

1. In which direction are you now heading?

2. If you started out going north and you didn't make a U-turn, would you be headed in the right direction?

3. If your favorite lake were to the north instead of the south, and you followed the rest of the turns as written above, in which direction would you ultimately be headed?

   TIP: *Are you creating a mental map? Or perhaps imagining a compass dial moving with each turn? See if either helps work out the correct answers.*

Exercise 3

Without using paper, solve the following word problem: You're heading east toward Walt Disney World. In order to see a national monument, you take a right turn, then take two left turns, then cross a bridge, and then take a right turn and two more left turns.

1. In which direction are you now heading?

2. If you stopped at the bridge, which way would you be heading?

3. If instead of making two left turns (whenever indicated), you only made one left turn before continuing, which way would you be heading?

CONTINUED

SPATIAL RELATIONS *Continued*
Exercise 4

Without using paper, solve the following word problem: You're heading northeast toward a friend's house. They told you to stay on the main road for five miles, then take the next three right turns. When the road comes to a T, take a left, then two rights.

1. In which direction are you now heading?

2. If you made a U-turn instead of the first right turn, which way would you be heading?

Exercise 5

Without using paper, solve the following word problem: You're heading southwest to try a new burrito shop. You take a left to pick up some paper plates before heading in the opposite direction.

1. After two rights and another left, in which direction are you now heading?

2. If the burrito shop were located to the north (instead of southwest), which way would you end up heading after following the directions through step 1?

3. If the burrito shop were located to the south (instead of southwest), which way would you end up heading after following the directions through step 1?

MENTAL MATH

Exercise 1

Without using paper or a calculator, solve the following word problem: A baker takes three trays, each containing a dozen muffins, out of the oven to cool. But they discover the muffins at the corners of the pan have burned for all except one pan.

1. How many unburned muffins remain for the baker to sell?

2. If an additional two muffins in the middle of each tray were burned, how many remain salable?

3. If the customer doesn't mind burnt muffins, how many can be sold?

Exercise 2

Without using paper or a calculator, solve the following word problem: A father is 30 years older than his daughter but six years younger than his brother. His daughter is 12 years older than his brother's youngest child. His brother's youngest child is eight years old. How old is the father?

Exercise 3

Without using paper or a calculator, solve the following word problem: An orange tree has four branches with five oranges on each branch. A bird pecks down three oranges, and two people pick three oranges each. How many oranges remain?

CONTINUED

MENTAL MATH *Continued*
Exercise 4

Without using paper or a calculator, solve the following word problem: You're throwing a party and inviting 9 guests. One guest asks if his sister can come and bring her three roommates. You have six chairs and three benches that seat two people each. Do you have enough seats for everyone if you accept his request?

Exercise 5

Without using paper or a calculator, solve the following word problem: Six ducks walk into a field where 12 mice and four snakes live. The snakes eat one mouse each for breakfast each day. How many pairs of footprints would you expect to see in the field at sunset on the third day?

CARD WORK

Exercise 1

Lay out four playing cards faceup in a line. Study them for 30 seconds, then flip them facedown.

Now recall them in order of suit: spades, hearts, diamonds, then clubs (e.g., 1, 3, 4 of spades, Jack and King of hearts, etc.). Increase the number of cards for an added challenge.

Exercise 2

Lay out four playing cards faceup in a line. Study them for 30 seconds, then flip them facedown.

Now recall them in order from smallest to largest. Increase the number of cards for an added challenge.

Exercise 3

Lay out five playing cards faceup in two lines, one over the other (a 2-by-3 grid). Study them for 30 seconds, then flip them facedown.

Now recall them, starting in the top left corner and moving clockwise, skipping over every other card (in an alternating fashion) until you've named all the cards. Increase the number of cards by increments of 2 cards (to keep an odd number of cards) for an added challenge.

Exercise 4

Lay out five playing cards faceup in a pentagon/circle layout. Study them for 30 seconds, then flip them facedown.

Start by recalling the top card, then move to the bottom right card, then back up to the upper left card; and continue as if you were drawing a star between the numbers.

CONTINUED

Exercise 5

Lay out eight playing cards faceup, forming a grid two cards high and four cards wide. Study the bottom row for 30 seconds, then flip those cards facedown (leaving the top row faceup).

Starting with the upper left card, recall the cards in a crisscross manner, switching between faceup and facedown cards (like lacing a shoe). Increase the number of cards for an added challenge. See if you can use the cards in the top row as cues to remember the cards in the bottom row (e.g., same number or suit).

STRATEGY CHECK: ORDER UP!

Read the list of the following items for one minute. Then turn the page so you can't see the items and see how many you can recall without looking.

Beth	Orange	Latte	Jude
Decaf	Medium	Mark	Small
Medium	Paul	Large	Double shot

Number of items	You're a great . . .	Because . . .
1 to 5	Barista	You've got the ingredients lined up for a great espresso drink.
6 to 10	Referee	You know who was where when that last penalty happened.
11 or 12	Teacher	You know the names of the kids in your class and probably the names of their parents, too. Rock on.

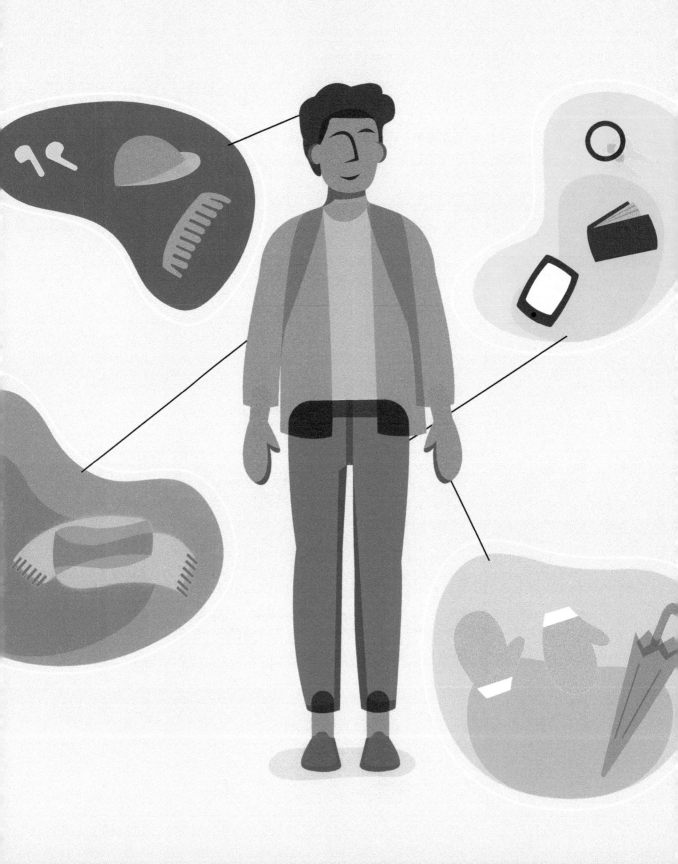

CHAPTER 4

REMEMBER THAT TIME?

(Long-Term Memory)

A good snapshot keeps a moment from running away.
—Eudora Welty

Long-term memory is our ability to hold on to information over long periods of time, for minutes, days, or even years. In our everyday lives, we rely on long-term memory to navigate both new and old situations. We apply our previously established knowledge of cooking to a new recipe (e.g., most cookies bake at 350 degrees Fahrenheit), but we can also navigate familiar situations using long-term memory, such as knowing which turn to take or where that speed trap is on the highway. Most activities that involve organizing and elaborating on information for later recall engage this type of memory.

Our memories become stronger when they are better organized and elaborated on more. Some lucky ducks have supreme long-term memories, a grace of genetics and life experience. The rest of us have to use some form of mental hustling to sharpen our memory. With those strategies in our pocket, we can feel more confident in conversation, more certain in our choices, and less dependent on notes or other memory aids. Compared to short-term and working memory, long-term memory persists despite the cessation of input or active rehearsal of information (e.g., repeating a phrase over and over in your head). Think of it like a basket: Once you drop a detail into your long-term memory basket, it stays there. To continue that analogy, we rely on working memory to take in information, kind of like a funnel that we feed into the basket; the bigger the funnel is, the more memories will land in the basket. (Keeping them in the basket is another thing, as is retrieving them from the basket.)

Formation of a long-term memory is strengthened through repetitive exposure to information, such as hearing a new acquaintance's name repeated over the course of a day. Additionally, certain emotionally charged or personally relevant information can often result in effective long-term memory formation, allowing it to be recalled the next day or years later after one exposure (e.g., hearing the results of a medical test or the name of a newborn family member). The formation of a long-term memory (scientifically called long-term potentiation) involves a series of changes in neurons (brain cells) as they communicate with one another. Much like plant roots growing toward the water and minerals in the soil, brain cells grow vast networks of interconnected brain cells in response to electrical impulses resulting from input from the world, like witnessing a sunset. Importantly, the changes in these brain cells rely on nutrients and minerals, such as calcium and amino acids, which we (hopefully) provide our body through nutritious meals or our body synthesizes using "ingredients" on hand.

Many of the strategies for recall amp up the electrical impulses by engaging various parts of the brain to reinforce or elaborate on newly learned information. For example, the body list described in chapter 1 ties new information to familiar body parts. Our mind already represents those body parts clearly, so mental visualization of a new-to-you bit of information alongside this familiar body part creates a stronger memory. Similarly, placing a time line of events across a familiar expanse, such as a football field or your own backyard, creates clarity in recall as you rely on the more established information to give context or meaning to the newly learned information. Additionally, use of detailed sensory information (like visualizing ice cream melting on your face) fires up the emotion centers of the brain, resulting in stronger memories.

MENTAL MAPS: BODY
Exercise 1

(1) Read through this prefilled body map while imagining each object on your own body in the same location. Use as much emotionally evocative detail as possible (e.g., roses growing out your nose, or stapling a book to your forehead), as this helps register it in memory. **(2)** See how many times you need to read through it before you can freely recall each of the items listed. **(3)** Wait 30 minutes and see how many you can recall. Note: Sometimes the items are placed strategically, such as rose on nose (because they rhyme and you smell roses with your nose).

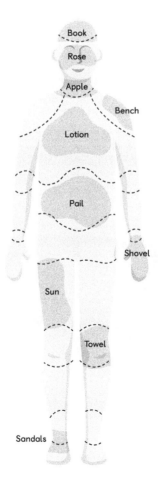

CONTINUED

MENTAL MAPS: BODY *Continued*

Exercise 2

Place the following ingredients onto your own body map. It can be the same as the previous activity or you can pick new body parts to map the following onto:

GREEN BEANS • RICE • SALT • OLIVE OIL • TOMATOES • WATER • ONION • CAPERS • BUTTER • SOY SAUCE

Recall after 20 minutes.

Exercise 3

Organize the following names alphabetically (in your head or on paper), then map them onto the body map of your choice:

FRANK • LOISE • PEDRO • BOB • CAROLYN • TENESHA • MORGAN • ZOEY • ISABELLA • BRIAN

Recall after 30 minutes.

> TIP: *To increase rememberability, visualize an emotionally-charged imaginary feature about each person related to where it is placed on the body map. E.g., to remember Collin, I might rhyme someone who needs to "call in" a robbery.*

Exercise 4

Organize the following bits of information by any method you choose, then put them on a body map of your choice:

TRAIN • CAN • LEMON • FROG • PILLOW • FORK • SHOE • NAPKIN • LAVENDER • BOLOGNA

Recall after one hour.

MENTAL MAPS: FLOOR PLAN

Instead of a body map, use locations (and objects) in your home or another familiar structure (e.g., kitchen table, living room rug) to organize the following information. Visualize in emotionally-charged detail the spaces where you "place" each object (e.g., melted cheese on the pillow case):

> TIRE · PARROT · CHEESE · BANDAGE · LIGHT BULB · GARBAGE BILL · FLOUR · SALVE

Write down each location and the bit of information it houses. Once you've done so, see how many pairings you can recall after one hour.

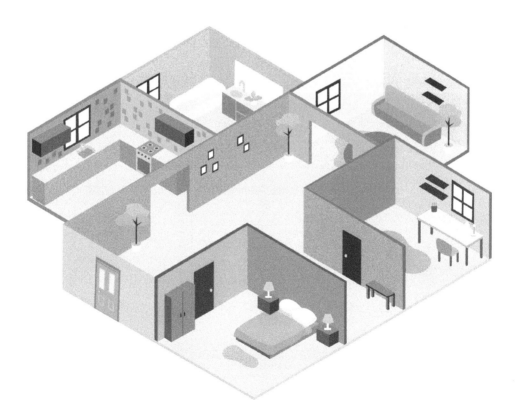

MENTAL MAPS: FIELDWORK
Exercise 1

Timing and sequence can be crucial. Place each of the following steps in the corresponding area of the field by number. Then rehearse the steps in the order they appear on the soccer field (or pull up another sports field/territory). Tie action/emotion to each step, such as dumping the water in step 3 onto the field over a player's head. See how many you recall after one hour.

1. Open the door.

2. Take down people's names.

3. Bring them water.

4. Interview people with names beginning with G.

5. Give the others paperwork.

6. Interview people with names beginning with K.

7. Call people with names beginning with B.

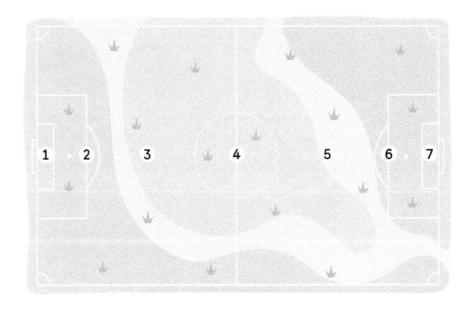

Exercise 2

The following is a list of remarkable women and crucial dates in their lives. Place the following women on the soccer field (or field of your choice) in order of the time line of their accomplishments. See what emotionally charged image you can create, such as Billie Jean King throwing her racket up in the air. Rehearse. See how many dates and details you can recall after one hour.

1. 1933: Frances Perkins becomes secretary of labor.

2. 1903: Marie Curie wins the Nobel Prize in Physics.

3. 1850: Harriet Tubman undertakes her first Underground Railroad mission.

4. 1917: Jeannette Rankin is sworn in as the first woman elected to Congress.

5. 1955: Rosa Parks sits down before the Montgomery bus boycott.

6. 1973: Billie Jean King wins the tennis match, "The Battle of the Sexes."

7. 1987: Aretha Franklin is inducted into the Rock and Roll Hall of Fame.

MENTAL MAPS: YOU CHOOSE
Exercise 1

Using the memory device of your choice, place the following holidays in order by earliest possible date and see how many you recall after one hour. Extra points if you can recall the dates in addition to the correct order. See which memory strategies you might use, such as emotionally-charged images or rhyming the date with a phrase.

1. **Día de Los Muertos:** November 1

2. **Christmas:** December 25

3. **Diwali:** October/November

4. **Chinese New Year:** late January/early February

5. **Hanukkah:** early to mid-December

6. **Nowruz (Persian New Year):** late March

7. **Bodhi Day:** usually January

Exercise 2

Memorize the following directions, using any method we have discussed so far. After 20 minutes, complete the maze on the next page to see if you've made it home or are stranded for the night.

1. Left
2. Right
3. Right
4. U-turn at end
5. Right
6. Left
7. Left
8. Right

Exercise 3

Memorize the following directions, using any method we have discussed so far. After 20 minutes, complete the maze on the next page to see if you've made it home or are stranded for the night.

1. Right
2. Second left
3. Left
4. Third left
5. Right
6. Right
7. Left

TIP: *For more practice, write out your own directions using the maze on the next page for reference and practice memorizing them or give them to a friend to memorize and find their way home.*

CONTINUED

Exercise 3 *Continued*

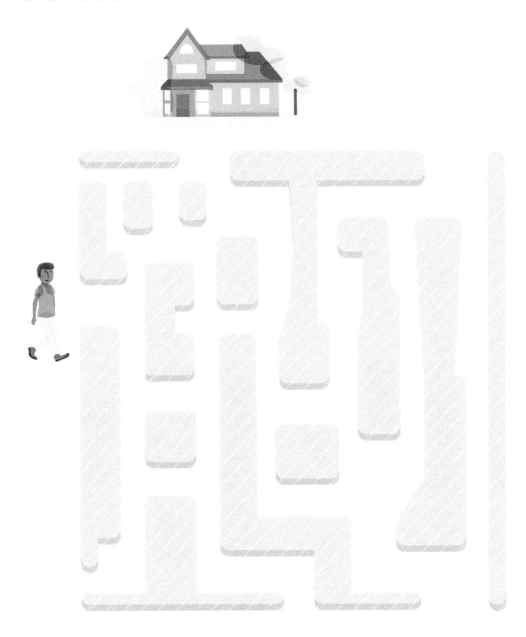

LINKING FEATURES
Exercise 1

Remembering names takes a bit of added effort. Find a feature on each of the following faces that helps you remember their name (e.g., Frank is a tank because of his strong chin line). See how many you can recall after 30 minutes:

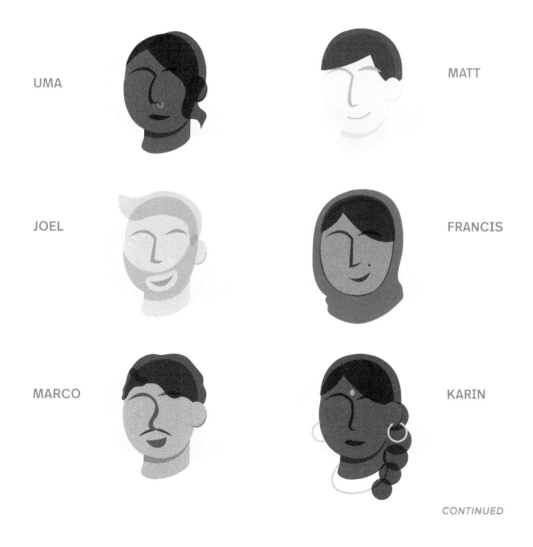

UMA

MATT

JOEL

FRANCIS

MARCO

KARIN

CONTINUED

LINKING FEATURES *Continued*
Exercise 2

Find a feature on each of the following animals that helps you remember their name (e.g., Spot has a spot on one eye). See how many you can recall after 30 minutes:

LUCKY

SHILOH

STAR

DRAKE

LULU

PETE

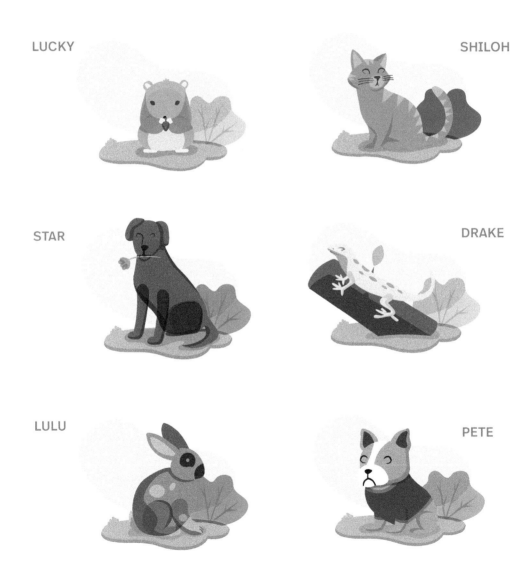

ELABORATE

We make associations to make remembering things easier. Elaboration is extending or adding to material, typically with information we already know. Here are some exercises in elaboration that use prompts for each word in the list to be remembered.

Exercise 1

Using your existing memories, answer the following prompts to elaborate on the following items (e.g., "NOTE" is similar to "letter"). Sometimes the prompts will be hard to think of an exact answer for, so just get as close as possible. See how many you can recall two hours later.

1. This word is similar to . . .

2. This word reminds me of . . .

3. This word sounds like (e.g., what the word sounds like or the sound it might make) . . .

APPLE · **REINDEER** · **FROG** · **TRACK** · **CREST** · **DRAWING** · **MOP** · **TRIP** · **RED**

Exercise 2

Using your existing memories, answer the following prompts to elaborate on the following items. See how many you can recall two hours later.

1. The word opposite of this is . . .

2. Someone I associate with this word is . . .

3. This word reminds me of the movie . . .

LAUGH · **TRADE** · **MISSION** · **SAD** · **CRIME** · **SHADE** · **COUGH** · **SHARP** · **PLOW**

CONTINUED

ELABORATE *Continued*

Exercise 3

Using your existing memories, answer the following prompts to elaborate on the following items. See how many you can recall two hours later.

> LARK · FREE · SPONTANEOUS · PILE · PLOT · SHAPE · MIDDLE · BEAR · BOX

1. A hand gesture I'd do to demonstrate this word is . . .

2. A food I associate with this word is . . .

3. This word reminds me of the character . . .

ALL THE DEETS

Exercise 1

Write out the instructions to your favorite card game. Be as thorough as possible. Now pick up a deck of cards and play the game based on the steps you wrote. See if you omitted details or recalled them all.

Exercise 2

Write out the instructions for how to make a cup of coffee in as much detail as possible. Give the instructions to someone and see if they can complete the task by doing only those steps as written.

TRIVIA RECALL

Exercise 1

Drawing on your memory of science and invention, answer the following questions. If you do not know the answer to any question, check the answer key. Then return in 24 hours and see if you remember them.

1. Who discovered gravity and when?

2. Who invented the motor-operated airplane?

3. What is the symbol for the chemical element gold?

4. When did the Iron Age begin?

Exercise 2

Drawing on your memory of food, answer the following questions. If you do not know the answer to any question, check the answer key. Then return in an hour and see if you remember them.

1. When was the invention of canning shared publicly?

2. When was chocolate first produced by humans?

3. When was the Food and Drug Administration founded?

4. When and where were food stamps launched?

CONTINUED

TRIVIA RECALL *Continued*

Exercise 3

Replace the capitalized word with another from the same category (e.g., HAMMER could be another tool, like screwdriver) for these famous book and movie titles:

1. A Few Good CHILDREN

2. AirBUS!

3. FIREFIGHTER Zhivago

4. Lady CAT

5. Close Encounters of the SIXTH Kind

6. BraveLEG

7. The Lord of the BRACELETS

8. PHANTOMbusters

9. Blazing YOKES

10. All the SENATOR'S Men

11. The BOBCAT King

Exercise 4

Replace the capitalized word with another from the same category (e.g., body part, flower) for these famous sayings:

1. A rolling SEDIMENT gathers no ORGANISMS.

2. A bad workman always blames his UTENSILS.

3. A bird in HEAD is worth two in the SHRUB.

4. Two MISSTEPS don't make a LEFT.

5. A chain is only as FLEXIBLE as its STIFFEST link.

6. Actions SMELL louder than LETTERS.

Exercise 5

Replace the capitalized word with another from the same category (e.g., body part, flower) for these common foods:

1. Fried green KUMQUATS

2. Cool as a POTATO

3. ANGELed eggs

4. Three PEA salad

5. HORSES in a blanket

6. Don't spill the POPPYSEEDS

7. Low-hanging SPOILS

8. ABC sandwich

9. All-you-can-INHALE

10. KNUCKLE pasta

11. CHERUB food cake

12. Swedish WHISKcakes

13. Don't LAUGH over spilled JUICE

CONTINUED

TRIVIA RECALL *Continued*

Exercise 6

Unscramble the letters to identify the celestial locale—if there is a space, then multiple words are in the answer (all letters stay within the word in which they are placed):

1. YKMLI   AWY

2. IERTJPU

3. UUASNR

4. UERYCRM

5. OSRION   BLTE

6. KLCAB   OEHL

7. RESUPNVAO

8. EOTMSC

9. ARSEIDTO

10. RLNUA   SPLICEE

Exercise 7

Unscramble the letters to identify the well-known scientist. If there is a space, then multiple words are in the answer (all letters stay within the word in which they are placed). If some (or many) are new to you, test your knowledge at a later date to see how many you can recall:

1. ERMAHSDIEC (Hint: "Eureka!")

2. DLEINA   UOLIENRLB (Hint: potential energy)

3. NEILS   HBOR (Hint: Quantum theory)

4. HRCLAE   AORSCN (Hint: *Silent Spring*)

5. EROGGE   TIHOGASWNN   ECRRAV (Hint: soil depletion)

6. ERONELFC   ETNNGLIAHIG (Hint: British nurse)

7. ISLUOANC   IRCOCPEUSN (Hint: center of the universe)

8. IREMA   IUCER (Hint: radioactivity)

9. ELSCRHA   NWIADR (Hint: Galapagos)

10. EREN   SECTDEASR (Hint: " . . . therefore I am")

11. LNSAIDOR   NNIKARFL (Hint: DNA)

12. JNEA   OLOADLG (Hint: chimps)

13. CPHIETSOPRA (Hint: medicine)

14. YOHODTR   VANGUHA (Hint: NASA)

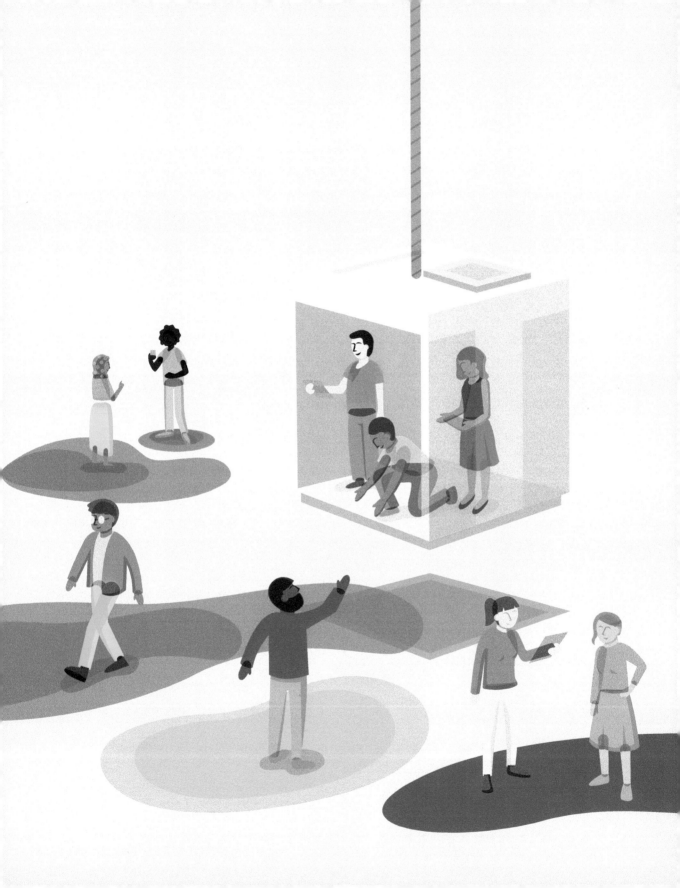

CHAPTER 5

PUTTING IT ALL TOGETHER

(Executive Functioning)

We cannot keep all of the details of the world in our brains, so we use models to simplify the complex into understandable and organizable chunks.
—Shane Parrish & Rhiannon Beaubien

When you think about executive functioning (EF), as earlier stated, think of a corporate executive and all the activities they engage in, from monitoring progress to strategizing the next big move. Similarly, your executive abilities allow you to move through the world in an organized fashion, adjusting course as needed based on feedback from your environment. We often rely on external devices to assist us with our EF, such as digital or manual calendars, alerts, and planners. EF is often conceptualized as applying previously acquired knowledge to novel situations; for example, you might use your knowledge of knots to figure out how to make a secure rope ladder or how to untie a knot using deductive reasoning. Working memory is often thought of as a subtype of EF, whereas long-term memory is more distinct (though it relies on EF strategies for effective uptake, storage, and retrieval of information).

Another type of memory that relies heavily on EF is prospective memory (PM), which (as the name suggests) means remembering something in the future. This could be in response to a cue in the environment (e.g., stop when you see a red light) or a certain point in time (e.g., take your medication at 7 p.m. daily). PM can be focal (related to the task at hand) or nonfocal (not directly related to the process at hand). Remembering to hit the brakes at a stop sign is focal, whereas remembering to mark a tally each time you say the word "the" while singing a song is not focal (or not directly related to the process of singing). The nonfocal PM task requires a substantial amount of monitoring in order to execute it accurately, which is where EF comes in. Again, this is why we rely on the many ways of automating responses to such nonfocal cues through the use of timers, software programs, and location-based smartphone alerts. How do we know when to apply our old knowledge to novel situations? When do we think "out of the box"? These are questions for our EF. When do we change our approach in response to feedback versus persisting in the same way? If you were driving down a highway and heard there would be a tornado 30 miles later, you'd need to reroute (not a tough decision). For more tricky decisions, such as how to find time in your daily schedule to go shopping between meetings, you'll likely need to use more executive strategies, like prioritizing, delegating, multitasking, and projecting time estimates and resource management.

Next, you'll find exercises in reasoning, monitoring of attention and task progress, organizing information, and more. When we become savvier with EF, we can take on more tasks without sacrificing effectiveness, or we can simply bask in the freed-up time and energy of implementing an effective EF strategy, such as setting a timer instead of watching the clock.

MOVING PARTS

Exercise 1

An elevator holds four people and travels from floor one to five. There are 25 people on the first floor. Three people are afraid of heights and don't want to travel higher than the third floor. What is the fewest number of trips (up and back down = 1) needed to get five people to each floor? (Tip: Use scratch paper, draw the floors, and circle groups or cross out people as you go.)

Exercise 2

A harbor holds 10 large boats and five smaller boats. At the mouth of the harbor, a large and small boat can pass at the same time, or two large boats can pass, or three small boats can pass. Any other combination will be too wide. What is the fewest number of crossings through the mouth of the harbor needed to take all boats out to sea?

Exercise 3

The mouth of a harbor is wide enough that one large and one small boat can pass at the same time, two large boats can pass, and three small boats can pass. Any other combination will be too wide. What is the fewest number of crossings needed to take all boats out to sea if the harbor contains 12 small boats and six large boats that need to leave for the day?

CONTINUED

MOVING PARTS *Continued*

Exercise 4

An elevator holds three people and travels from floor one to six. There are 30 people on the first floor. Ten people are claustrophobic and won't travel with more than one other person. What is the fewest number of trips (up and back down = 1) needed to get five people to each floor?

Exercise 5

The mouth of a harbor is wide enough that a large and small boat can pass each other, but two large boats must go end to end, and two small boats can pass each other. Any other combination will be too wide. What is the fewest number of crossings needed to take all boats out to sea if the harbor contains four small boats and 10 large boats that need to leave for the day?

HIGHLIGHTS

Exercise 1

Count the number of times these letters appear in the same order (with or without separating spaces/symbols): THE

The town's mayor let Herman provide the opening speech for the season, knowing he could breathe easy, as he found Herman to be someone he liked versus the person he loathed.

Exercise 2

Count the number of times these letters appear in the same order (with or without separating spaces/symbols): MOR

Given Morticia's many talents, she wasn't sure if she should sing to them or tell them original ghost stories from Oregon Trail adventures she had over last term or make origami armor.

Exercise 3

Count the number of times these letters appear in the same order (with or without separating spaces/symbols): AL

The many wallflowers at the party felt all right on the periphery of the dance hall, even though friends were calling them all to come waltz on the smooth walnut floor.

CONTINUED

Exercise 4

Count the number of times these letters appear in the same order (with or without separating spaces/symbols): REN

The children rendered the arena's resounding applause siren-like in intensity, while parents, entrenched in the bustling crowds of renowned cartoon characters, renounced ever returning to the hectic scene.

Exercise 5

Count the number of times these letters appear in the same order (with or without separating spaces/symbols): LAN

The clan's slanted planks came down with a clank, which left the lane covered in planks—and the flanking land the only place where the clan could plan to pass in their clamorous cars.

MENTAL PIVOTS

Exercise 1

Read through the following lines. Every time you encounter "ER," begin reading letters in the reverse direction (right to left or vice versa). Once you've reversed on an "ER," you won't reverse on it again (just read it like any other set of letters). Count how many times you change directions.

1. ABREQLSERNSLRSESREDFLMESRSREPFERFRAMLO

2. OPREAFDELSREFAMERSAFELASREAFAPERAPRAELQ

3. SLAEFREFALWERANARELENARAMWOEPTARENLSOAR

4. RESEEFLATRERAWREEREERRERERREEEERRRERЕREE

5. REELFSRDEERFRRREOOPRSEEERSLFWBREOLERWLREWMER

6. RELSMFSKERRRALSRESFSLERSAEAREALFERRESLFEERALSR

Exercise 2

Read through the following lines. Every time you encounter "RI," begin reading letters in the reverse direction. Once you've reversed on an "RI," you won't reverse on it or either of the letters involved again (just read it like any other set of letters). Count how many times you change directions.

1. ABIRQLSRINSLRSESIRDFLMESRSIRPFRIFRAMLO

2. AEFIRFLWRIANAIRLENARAMWOEPTAIRNLSIAR

3. OPIRAFDELSIRFAMRISAFELASIRAFAPRIAPRAELQ

4. IRSEEFLATRRIAWIRRIEIRRIIIREERIRROIRIER

5. IRELFSRDERIFIRRIROOPRSEERISLFWBIROLRIWLIRWMRI

6. IRLSMFSKRIRRALSIRSFSLRISAEAIRALFRIIRSLFERIALSR

Putting It All Together **73**

MENTAL PIVOTS *Continued*

Exercise 3

Read through the following lines. Every time you encounter "OA," begin reading letters in the reverse direction. Once you've reversed on an "OA," you won't reverse on it again (just read it like any other set of letters). Count how many times you change directions.

1. ABREQLAORNSLROASREDFLAOSRSREOAERFRAMLO

2. OPAOEAFDEOASRAOMEOARSAAOSFLOASRAPRAE

3. SLAEFREFALWERANARELENARAMWAOEPTARENLSOAR

4. ELFSAODEOAERFAORRREOOOASEEERSLFWBREOLERWOAL

5. ASDLVAOPRGNLSKFOAANWGADLKAOMBNDEROALSASOFA

Exercise 4

Read through the following lines. Every time you encounter "WN," begin reading letters in the reverse direction. Once you've reversed on a "WN," you won't reverse on it again (just read it like any other set of letters). Count how many times you change directions.

1. ABRENWWNSERNWSLWENSRNWERFRWNAMLO

2. EAFDNWELSWNREFAMWSNWAFEWNLNWERAPWRMN

3. ALNWERAWNARELENARAMWOENWPTARENWLWR

4. ASLVMWFNWLATRWNASDLKFEERNWSWNDLFKWNREE

5. OPNWRRNNRALWNSRESNWERSLWNWNNNWNWWWWWNEER

Exercise 5

Read through the following lines. Every time you encounter "SK," begin reading letters in the reverse direction. Once you've reversed on an "SK," you won't reverse on it again (just read it like any other set of letters). Count how many times you change directions.

1. NWERFKSRWNAASDSKLFKJSDAFLKSAJSDFLSKMKLKO

2. ALKSFJSALDSSKFJSSDAKFJAKSDLKFDSKVKLMNZSSSKXCV

3. ZMXCKSLVPQEWTUIADGSLIUEPZXVLIJZZMXSKNCVQER

4. ZMXCVNAPQIOERTJLKSDFGKSZMDFSKNVEQRGI

5. PQUEKSWRTLKSDJGZXCVMWEGSKJDFPGOULKSDSGHSKQP

6. KSSSSSSKOMXPKSXPDKSLPWJZVKZZPLSSKDPKSLCXVOIZKS

STRATEGY CHECK (LONG-TERM MEMORY)

Draw on your memory to see how many birthdays you can recall. Feel free to include family, friends, pets, nations, and companies—really dig in.

1 to 10	BFF	You know your pals. True blue.
11 to 20	Friendly Traveler	You have an eye on history and current affairs.
21 plus	Savoir Faire Soul	You know the deets on your dinner partner, their pet, and when they founded their business. Sláinte!

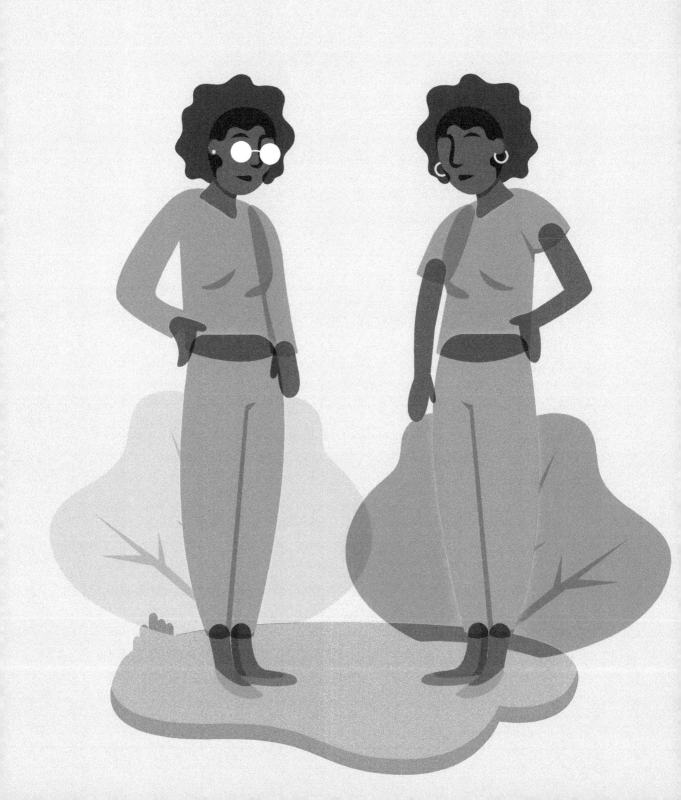

CHAPTER 6

HEY, WHAT'S THAT—AND THAT?!

(Attention and Flexibility)

Pay attention to your attention.
—Unknown

I like the phrase "pay attention" because it signifies that, like money, our attention is precious; we spend it on various things, so we might as well be picky. Interestingly, our beliefs about our ability to pay attention influence how well we pay attention to things. So many things vie for our attention these days. Much of the media we consume is composed of short bursts of attention-grabbing material meant to be processed briefly in small chunks (think social media or news headlines). We often don't have to work too hard for the next object of our attention, though the quality of that next target may not be high. As a result, we often feel scattered as our attention jumps from one subject to the other. In contrast to brief and shallow attention, our ability to hold our focus on one target (sustained attention) is something we have to make a special effort to cultivate. Some of us get squirmy and bored, especially during repetitive tasks. One trick is to find ways to reinforce (or reward) continued engagement, perhaps by reminding ourselves of our overarching goal/purpose, reviewing progress thus far, or taking quick breaks to refresh our minds.

What stops us from sustaining attention? Typically, it's a "Squirrel!" moment when our interest is waning and something else pops into our mind or field of view, like a video on the side of our computer screen that has the most intriguing photo preview. Twenty minutes later, we realize we're no nearer to our goal. (Though hopefully we've had a good laugh or learned a fun, new fact at least.) There is a lot of information out there, so our ability to select what we pay attention to (selective attention) becomes extremely valuable. It also helps if we minimize distractions, such as having a clear desk, not facing a window overlooking a busy scene, and turning off random alerts from various electronics.

Additionally, the processing of information for a higher level of detail (e.g., ensuring emails are typo-free and include necessary explanations) is again something that can require your special attention and is not particularly supported by our everyday environments. It's not about making *zero* errors, per se, but more about figuring out how you can organize tasks such that you make errors less often and catch them more quickly when you do. A key to doing this is reducing *cognitive overhead*, or the number of "logical connections or jumps your brain has to make in order to understand or contextualize the thing you're looking at," as described by web designer and engineer David Demaree. Switching among tasks creates a mental penalty, so the less complex the things you switch among are, the less mental penalty you experience (e.g., switching among reading complex book passages versus among appliances you're cleaning). In the following activities, you'll engage your attention to detail/selective attention, attention switching or multitasking, and sustained attention. See which ways help reduce your cognitive overhead and optimize your abilities in these areas. Keep in mind the truth behind the myth of multitasking: You're nearly always going to be more effective by focusing on one task at a time, especially if a task is complex.

FEATURE RECALL

Exercise 1

Spot the differences between these two illustrations. Some differences are large, while others are small:

TIP: *For an added challenge, study the graphic on the top first, then cover it up and see how many differences you can spot without looking back at the first graphic.*

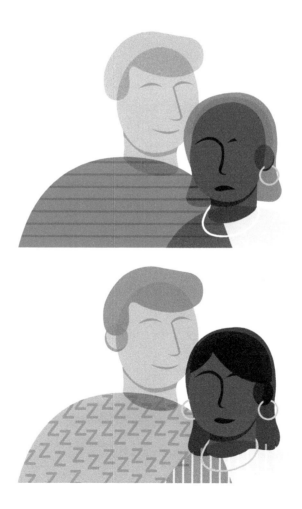

CONTINUED

FEATURE RECALL *Continued*

Exercise 2

Spot the differences between these two illustrations. Some differences are large, while others are small:

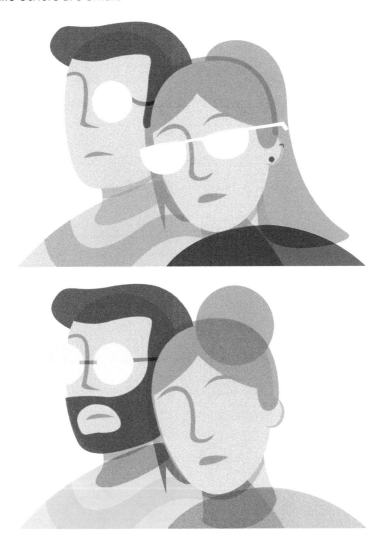

Exercise 3

Spot the differences between these two illustrations. Some differences are large, while others are small:

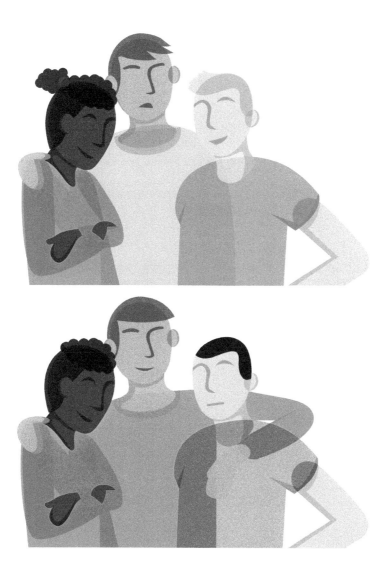

CONTINUED

FEATURE RECALL *Continued*

Exercise 4

Spot the differences between these two illustrations. Some differences are large, while others are small:

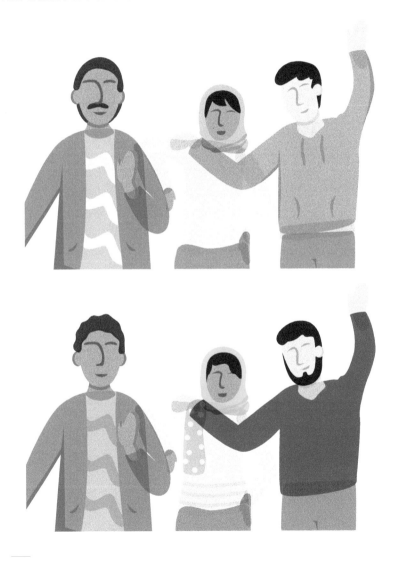

Exercise 5

Spot the differences between these two illustrations. Some differences are large, while others are small:

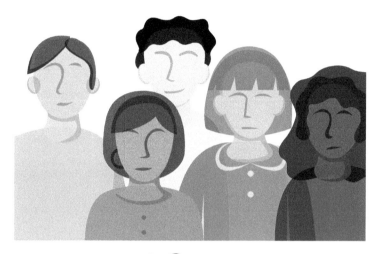

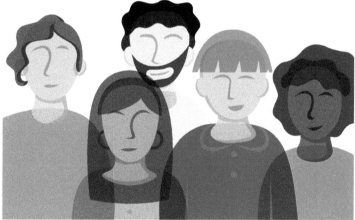

MULTITASKING
Exercise 1

Word Weaving: Switch between spelling a word from the first column backward and then naming an item from the second. Look away and spell the word from memory, or for support, glance or stare at the page while spelling. For an added challenge, time yourself and repeat at a much later time (or else you'll remember the answers—see if you can beat your previous time!).

Spell backward	Name the baby version of each animal:
Humor	Cat
Payment	Goat
Tongue	Pig
Standard	Horse
Health	Dog
Touch	Bird
Winding	Kangaroo
Whistle	Sheep
Nation	Goose

Exercise 2

Repeat for the following lists:

Spell backward	Name the continent in which each country is located:
Wagon	India
Chair	Canada
Puddle	Indonesia
Card stock	Angola
Button	France
Blanket	Brazil
Thermometer	Madagascar
Bottle	Algeria
Doorknob	Iran

CONTINUED

MULTITASKING *Continued*
Exercise 3

Repeat for the following lists:

Spell backward	Name the missing part of each fairy tale name:
Cheyanne	Jack and _____
Theresa	Little Red _____ _____
Ada	Hansel and _____
Evie	The Tortoise and the _____
Kaitlyn	Three Little _____
Estrella	Cinder____
Miriam	Snow White and the _____ _____
Alexandria	Rumpel _____
Dayana	The Princess and the _____

Exercise 4

Repeat for the following lists:

Spell backward	Name a dish containing . . .
Snowboarding	Cinnamon
Boxing	Jalapeños
Ice hockey	Flour
Baseball	Cream
Skiing	Maple syrup
Rollerblading	Onions
Surfing	Marshmallows
Ultimate Frisbee	Black olives
Cricket	Spinach

MENTAL COMPARISONS

Exercise 1

Rank the following peppers in order from spiciest to mildest. If you do not know the rankings already, check the answer key. Then return in an hour and see if you remember them.

1. Habanero
2. Chipotle
3. Devil's Tongue
4. Pepperoncini
5. Tabasco
6. Serrano
7. Poblano
8. Carolina Cayenne
9. Bell pepper
10. Jalapeño

Exercise 2

Reorder the following items in order from longest to shortest:

TIP: Pay special attention to detail on this one so you don't mistake one size for another.

1. Great blue shark: slightly less than 1.5 times the length of the oceanic whitetip shark
2. Whitetip shark: half the length of the great blue shark
3. Great white shark: four times longer than the blacktip shark
4. Nurse shark: just shy of two times the length of the whitetip shark
5. Thresher shark: three times longer than the blacktip shark

6. Oceanic whitetip shark: slightly more than 1.5 times longer than the whitetip shark

7. Hammerhead shark: slightly more than two times longer than the blacktip shark

8. Blacktip shark: slightly less than half the length of the nurse shark

Exercise 3

Reorder the following items in order from largest to smallest based on land area. Try it from memory, then reattempt at a later date after learning the correct sizes/order:

1. Minnesota: slightly smaller than Utah

2. Oregon: basically six times smaller than Alaska

3. Montana: slightly more than 1.5 times the size of Oregon

4. Arizona: slightly more than 1⅓ times the size of Utah

5. Alaska: more than two times larger than Texas

6. Nevada: slightly more than 1⅓ times the size of Minnesota

7. Utah: slightly more than half the size of California

8. New Mexico: slightly more than 1.5 times the size of Minnesota

9. Texas: a bit more than 1.5 times the size of California

10. California: slightly less than two times the size of Minnesota

11. Michigan: slightly less than half the size of Arizona

CONTINUED

MENTAL COMPARISONS *Continued*
Exercise 4

Reorder the following planets from smallest to largest:

1. Saturn: nine times larger than Earth

2. Venus: only slightly smaller than Earth

3. Earth

4. Neptune: only slightly smaller than Uranus

5. Mars: about half the size of Earth

6. Jupiter: 11 times larger than Earth

7. Mercury: about a third of the size of Earth

8. Uranus: four times larger than Earth

Exercise 5

Reorder the following sports by their number of global fans (most to least fans, per SportsShow.net):

1. Cricket: 2.5 times tennis

2. Basketball: 4.4 times baseball

3. Rugby: slightly less than half of table tennis

4. Table tennis: just shy of volleyball

5. Field hockey: four times baseball

6. Volleyball: just a bit less than two times baseball

7. Soccer: 3.5 times more than tennis

8. Baseball: half of tennis

9. Tennis: half of field hockey

10. American football: equal to rugby

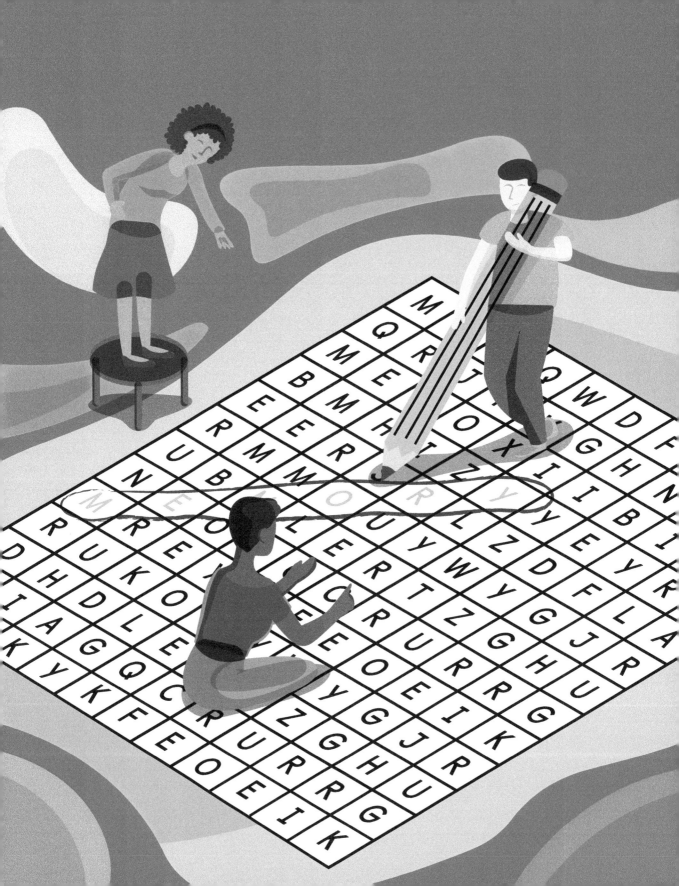

CHAPTER 7

CHECK THE CLOCK

(Processing Speed)

I'm in a hurry, so let's do it slow once.
—A new take on an old saying

Processing speed is used during all kinds of tasks throughout our day. We employ it when we take in our surroundings after walking through the door or while driving and reacting quickly. Most of what we do requires a blend of prioritizing accuracy or speed. Generally, we know when to take all the time needed to make sure we file our taxes accurately (prioritizing accuracy) and when to skim an article in *People* magazine (prioritizing speed). But sometimes our time runs short, and we find that we didn't lock the car door or we end up paying $46 for that utility instead of $64 and now there's a late fee. It's quite difficult to improve both speed and accuracy at the same time, but with practice and good strategies, it can be possible to progress a little more quickly while maintaining or even improving accuracy. Here's an example of what such a strategy might look like: You're searching through a large amount of information and you want to do so both accurately and quickly, so you break it down into small chunks that are more manageable.

Processing speed is most relevant to the intake stage of memory and aspects of consolidation. Some people with slower processing speed might have trouble immediately recalling details. However, after some delay, they may find that more of what they learned earlier becomes accessible to them. (This is related to the time it takes to consolidate that information into accessible memory.) Another component of processing speed and general cognitive performance is emotion. When most people undertake tasks involving processing speed (i.e., time constraints), they have at least a mild tightening in their stomach, if not full-on anxiety, as their mind panics slightly from the pressure of time constraints. This is why relaxation strategies, such as belly breathing or grounding exercises, can be particularly helpful in calming your mind and bringing the critical thinking parts of your brain back online. What do I mean by online? As the psychiatrist Dr. Dan Siegel popularized, "flipping your lid" is when our mind becomes stressed by some situation and prioritizes the more primal parts of our brain in an effort to keep us alive, while deprioritizing the parts of the brain responsible for abstract thinking (our neocortex), making it difficult to think deeply or creatively. This is why test-taking can be so difficult at times; the combination of time constraints and high stakes (like your class grade or passing a licensing exam) stresses people out. But time constraints are just one piece of the puzzle. If you can approach timed tasks with some emotional intelligence and cognitive finesse, you're likely to do your best. Next are some activities that aim to engage your processing speed faculty and give you an opportunity to use strategies of chunking, visual organization, and pattern recognition while staying cool as a cucumber in a warm summer breeze.

THINK FAST

Exercise 1

List a color for every letter of the alphabet in five minutes. (It's harder than it sounds.) Make use of paint or crayon colors. If doing so with a friend, you can vote on the acceptability of any "creative" name colors.

_____

_____

_____

_____

Exercise 2

List a food for every letter of the alphabet in five minutes. Think of spices, fruits, or names of dishes or cuisines.

_____

_____

_____

_____

_____

CONTINUED

Exercise 3

List a city for every letter of the alphabet in 10 minutes. Consider places around the world. If needed, you can pull on fictional cities from movies or literature.

Exercise 4

List a type or name of a plant for every letter of the alphabet in 10 minutes. This could include trees, flowers, bushes, etc.

Exercise 5

List items you use with your hands (e.g., use, wear, or operate with your hand/hands) for every letter of the alphabet in 10 minutes. This could entail bathroom items, tools, kitchen items, etc.

READY, AIM, MARK!

In the following word search, see how many words from the list you can find in 60 seconds. Read through the list of words, then hit the timer.

Exercise 1

Time Tracker

```
K   M   H   D   E   L   A   Y   H   P
T   Z   Y   I   S   T   V   F   I   A
P   R   E   S   E   N   T   C   W   U
F   N   A   W   C   A   B   L   A   S
D   U   R   H   O   F   E   O   T   E
A   Y   T   O   N   T   F   C   C   A
Y   X   J   U   D   E   O   K   H   R
K   I   I   R   R   R   R   Q   B   L
M   O   N   T   H   E   E   Q   Z   Y
U   V   P   Q   M   I   N   U   T   E
```

after	delay	minute	second
before	early	month	watch
clock	future	pause	year
day	hour	present	

Exercise 2

Birding

```
I  Y  V  I  N  G  D  L  A  E
F  Q  F  U  F  S  U  O  V  R
R  L  B  D  L  T  C  O  I  O
O  C  O  K  O  T  K  N  A  O
B  H  O  C  T  V  U  Q  R  K
I  I  F  T  K  W  E  R  Y  R
N  C  L  R  W  I  N  G  E  A
F  K  H  L  Y  T  K  S  E  V
F  L  I  G  H  T  U  I  G  E
Y  M  I  G  R  A  T  E  G  N
```

aviary	duck	loon	rook
bill	egg	migrate	vulture
chick	flight	raven	wing
dove	flock	robin	

CONTINUED

READY, AIM, MARK! *Continued*

Exercise 3

Ahoy, Sailor!

```
B  B  M  C  G  J  S  A  S  O
O  O  A  A  C  W  T  A  C  K
W  O  S  P  L  I  L  T  K  F
S  M  T  S  I  N  P  R  A  E
T  S  H  I  N  D  O  I  B  N
E  H  C  Z  E  W  R  M  E  D
R  E  L  E  S  A  T  G  A  E
N  E  E  Z  E  R  U  A  M  R
Q  T  W  I  T  D  X  W  N  H
P  S  T  I  L  L  E  R  P  S
```

abeam	clew	port	tiller
boom	fender	sheets	trim
bow	lines	stern	windward
capsize	mast	tack	

Exercise 4

Herbs and Spices

```
G  I  N  G  E  R  N  F  D  R
R  S  A  F  F  R  O  N  I  S
S  R  C  H  E  R  V  I  L  V
V  O  T  F  E  N  N  E  L  A
N  S  R  B  C  H  I  L  I  N
U  E  P  A  R  S  L  E  Y  I
T  M  T  S  C  U  M  I  N  L
M  A  F  I  T  H  Y  M  E  L
E  R  T  L  A  N  I  S  E  A
G  Y  G  Y  C  H  I  V  E  S
```

anise	cumin	ginger	saffron
basil	chili	nutmeg	thyme
chervil	dill	parsley	vanilla
chives	fennel	rosemary	

CONTINUED

Exercise 5

Weather

```
H  Q  B  Y  I  N  Y  L  S  M
O  D  D  T  C  S  H  A  D  E
T  E  R  R  M  L  N  I  W  R
T  C  A  I  Y  V  O  U  E  A
O  W  H  I  Z  C  F  U  T  I
R  I  C  I  S  Z  S  R  D  N
N  N  L  H  L  F  L  N  V  S
A  D  E  A  E  L  X  E  O  L
D  Y  A  I  E  T  Y  Q  Z  W
O  T  R  L  T  S  T  O  R  M
```

chilly	dry	shade	tornado
clear	hail	sleet	wet
clouds	hot	snow	windy
drizzle	rain	storm	

Exercise 6

Flowers

```
A R T E M I S I A G F U I J P
V N R M A R I G O L D D H V A
I N H O N E Y S U C K L E K N
N S C C L E M A T I S D Z N S
C K I K F W O B M S W A N E Y
A C O R E O P S I S X H E C N
J P K G Y K P Q A N B L S A A
Y V V A L Z T R C H J I C T S
B C G I U Y B E I C B A A M T
P H L I L A C U H M H B B I U
M O R N I N G G L O R Y I N R
O T X H B H G T H Z T O O T T
X C F J K A L L I U M U S D I
U W I S T E R I A T P X A E U
Y B G Y T S I B Q M T V L M M
```

allium	coreopsis	marigold	primrose
artemisia	dahlia	morning glory	scabiosa
catmint	honeysuckle	nasturtium	vinca
clematis	lilac	pansy	wisteria

THE ODD ONES OUT

Exercise 1

Each word in the following list of sports isn't quite right (i.e., it has extra or out-of-place letters or is otherwise misspelled). Circle any out-of-place letters or cross out any extra/wrong letters. See how many you can correctly mark in 30 seconds.

1. Tracke
2. Bauxing
3. Ultimmate Frissbee
4. Competittive swimminng
5. Rownig
6. Waffle ball
7. Roller dirby
8. Crewe
9. Poool
10. Waightlifting
11. Galf
12. Serfing
13. Crecket
14. Snowboarrding
15. Chearleading
16. Footboll
17. Rugbey
18. Baiseball
19. Scateboarding
20. Tennise

Exercise 2

Each word in the following list of European self-governed domains and countries isn't quite right. Circle or cross out the letter (or letters) that is out of place. See how many you can correctly mark in 30 seconds.

1. Jerseey
2. Faroe Islandz
3. Monacoe
4. Vatican Citey
5. Isle of Mane
6. Mallta
7. Estoniea
8. Sloveinia
9. Switserland
10. Bulgeria
11. Belarous
12. Sweeden
13. Liecchtenstein
14. Albaniea
15. Portougal
16. Icelend
17. Belgeum
18. Spayin
19. Jermany
20. Finnland

Exercise 3

Each animal in the following list isn't quite right. Circle or cross out the letter (or letters) that are out of place. See how many you can correctly mark in 30 seconds.

1. Bummblebee
2. Musc deer
3. Ellk
4. Beever
5. Hoge
6. Crikket
7. Gireffe
8. Miink
9. Eagle ouwl
10. Lovebirrd
11. Dung beatle
12. Thornny devil
13. Buill
14. Wildkat
15. Whaile
16. Phig
17. Shreww
18. Haire
19. Quaail
20. Jagwuar

Exercise 4

Each household item in the following list isn't quite right. Circle or cross out the out-of-place letter or letters. See how many you can correctly mark in 30 seconds.

1. Pensil
2. Bhag
3. Bukmark
4. Waiste bin
5. Eyelineer
6. Lampshayde
7. Guetar
8. Rhug
9. Owtlet
10. Wather bottel
11. Monihtor
12. USB draive
13. Legh warmers
14. Speackers
15. Slippper
16. Bottel cap
17. Mirrror
18. Soufa
19. Plastik fork
20. Magneht

STRATEGY CHECK

See how quickly you can draw out the following message by ignoring all the numbers, capital letters, Zs, Ps, and Bs:

283AzPpcp4Zhe49b4p2e3JFrsP0p23tz99po98By0zop
P334uz940rh98Spe0alSDtbphw231e3a42l5t6h3984a3n6
34d3z45w34058i32s235bdp235o523bp3m235!0P

>60 seconds	Accuracy over speed can be a great tool!
31 to 60 seconds	Snappy!
11 to 30 seconds	Sign up for NASA!
<10 seconds	Are you sure you got the right message?

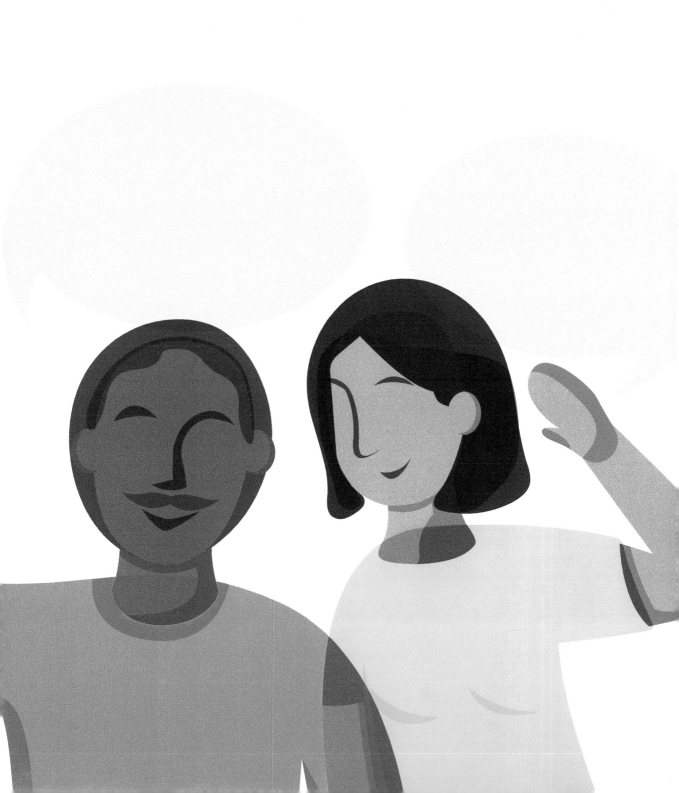

ANSWER KEY

CHAPTER 2

EYE-CATCHERS

Exercise 1 (page 17)

Photo: Eagle

1. **12, or 6 on each wing**
2. **Left**
3. **At an angle.**
4. **White/cream**
5. **Closed**

Exercise 2 (page 19)

Photo: Hockey

1. **3**
2. **Black, red, white, yellow, blue, and a tiny bit of green.**
3. **No**
4. **Yes**
5. **Blue and white**

Exercise 3 (page 21)

Photo: Building

1. **No**
2. **Red, orange, black, gray**
3. **5**
4. **No**

Exercise 4 (page 23)

Photo: Clocks

1. **45 and 60**
2. **3**
3. **2**
4. **12**
5. **6**

Exercise 5 (page 25)

Photo: Keyboard

1. **6, visibly**
2. **E, R, T, Y, U, A, S, D, F, G, H, J, Z, X, C, V, and B**
3. **3**
4. **1**
5. **4**

PALM READING

Exercise 1 (page 30)

1.

2.

Exercise 2 (page 31)

1.

2.

CHAPTER 3

CHUNKING

Exercise 2 (page 37)

Chunking suggestions: East/west; ending in "a" or not

Exercise 3 (page 37)

Chunking suggestions: sporting equipment and clothing items; smaller vs. larger items

Exercise 4 (page 37)

Chunking suggestions: first letter (A, B, F, or J); shorter vs. longer

SPATIAL RELATIONS

Exercise 1 (page 38)

1. Yes
2. No
3. Yes, but the dog will need to turn its head.

Exercise 2 (page 39)

1. South
2. No

3. North

Exercise 3 (page 39)

1. West
2. North

3. East

Exercise 4 (page 40)

1. Northeast

2. Southeast

Exercise 5 (page 40)

1. Northeast
2. South

3. North

Exercise 1 (page 41)

1. 28 muffins
2. 22 muffins

3. 36 muffins

Exercise 2 (page 41)
50 years old

Exercise 3 (page 41)
11 oranges

Exercise 4 (page 42)
No. Two more seats are needed. (You have 12 seats and 14 people will be there, including yourself.)

Exercise 5 (page 42)
6 pair (12 feet) since the snakes have eaten all the mice.

CHAPTER 4

TRIVIA RECALL

Exercise 1 (page 61)

1. Sir Isaac Newton (1687)
2. The Wright brothers (1903)
3. Au
4. 1200 BCE and 600 BCE, depending on the region

Exercise 2 (page 61)

1. 1810 by Nicolas Appert of France
2. As early as 1900 BCE by pre-Olmec cultures living in present-day Mexico
3. 1906
4. 1939 in Rochester, NY

Exercise 3 (page 62)

1. A Few Good Men
2. Airplane!
3. Doctor Zhivago
4. Lady Bird
5. Close Encounters of the Third Kind
6. Braveheart
7. The Lord of the Rings
8. Ghostbusters
9. Blazing Saddles
10. All the President's Men
11. The Lion King

Exercise 4 (page 63)

1. A rolling stone gathers no moss.
2. A bad workman always blames his tools.
3. A bird in hand is worth two in the bush.
4. Two wrongs don't make a right.
5. A chain is only as strong as its weakest link.
6. Actions speak louder than words.

Exercise 5 (page 63)

1. Fried green tomatoes
2. Cool as a cucumber
3. Deviled eggs
4. Three bean salad
5. Pigs in a blanket
6. Don't spill the beans
7. Low-hanging fruit
8. BLT sandwich
9. All-you-can-eat
10. Elbow pasta
11. Angel food cake
12. Swedish pancakes
13. Don't cry over spilled milk

Exercise 6 (page 64)

1. Milky Way
2. Jupiter
3. Uranus
4. Mercury
5. Orion's Belt
6. Black hole
7. Supernova
8. Comets
9. Asteroid
10. Lunar eclipse

Exercise 7 (page 65)

1. Archimedes
2. Daniel Bernoulli
3. Niels Bohr
4. Rachel Carson
5. George Washington Carver
6. Florence Nightingale
7. Nicolaus Copernicus
8. Marie Curie
9. Charles Darwin
10. René Descartes
11. Rosalind Franklin
12. Jane Goodall
13. Hippocrates
14. Dorothy Vaughan

CHAPTER 5

MOVING PARTS

Exercise 1 (page 69)

5: Only four floors need filling because the first floor is already brimming with people. You can move people at a rate of four per trip, so it will take five trips to move all 20 people to their respective floors. (You can leave the people who have a fear of heights on the first floor.)

Exercise 2 (page 69)

7: Four crossings of two large boats, two crossings of a large and small boat, and one crossing of three small boats.

Exercise 3 (page 69)

7: Three crossings of two large boats and four crossings of three smaller boats.

Exercise 4 (page 70)

10: Only five floors need filling; you can move people at a rate of three per trip for the first six trips/four floors (18 people). Then move two people per trip for the next two trips, and only one person for the last trip to fill the second floor. Five people will be left on the first floor.

Exercise 5 (page 70)

10: Six crossings of one large boat and four crossings of one large boat and one small boat.

HIGHLIGHTS

Exercise 1 (page 71)

7

Exercise 2 (page 71)

6

Exercise 3 (page 71)

7

Exercise 4 (page 72)

8

Exercise 5 (page 72)

10

MENTAL PIVOTS

Exercise 1 (page 73)

1.	4	**3.**	2	**5.**	8
2.	4	**4.**	12	**6.**	8

Exercise 2 (page 73)

1.	4	**3.**	4	**5.**	5
2.	2	**4.**	9	**6.**	8

Exercise 3 (page 74)

1.	4	**3.**	2	**5.**	4
2.	6	**4.**	5		

Exercise 4 (page 74)

1.	4	**3.**	2	**5.**	5
2.	4	**4.**	5		

Exercise 5 (page 75)

1.	4	**3.**	2	**5.**	4
2.	5	**4.**	2	**6.**	4

Exercise 1 (page 79)

From left to right:

The first person has different hair colors and different color/patterned shirts, and the top image is missing an ear.

The second person has different hair colors, different patterned shirts, different color necklaces, and different facial expressions; and the top image is missing an earring.

Exercise 2 (page 80)

From left to right:

The first person has different color shirts and different style glasses. The top image is clean shaven, and the bottom image has a beard.

The second person has different hairstyles and different color shirts, and the top image is wearing glasses and has two small earrings.

Exercise 3 (page 81)

From left to right:

The first person has different hairstyles, and the top image has a hair tie.

The second person has different hairstyles, different facial expressions, and different color shirts, and the top image is missing left arm.

The third person has different hairstyles/colors, different facial expressions, and different color shirts.

Exercise 4 (page 82)

From left to right:

The first person has different hairstyles and different color shirts, and the top image has a mustache.

The second person has different hairstyles and different style/color/patterned head scarves, and the bottom image has a shirt with stripes.

The third person has different hairstyles and different color sweatshirts; and the bottom image has a beard, and the sweatshirt has no drawstrings.

Exercise 5 (page 83)

From left to right:

The first person has different hairstyles and different color shirts.

The second person has different hairstyles and different color shirts, and the top image is missing an earring.

The third person has a beard in the bottom image.

The fourth person has different hairstyles, different facial expressions, and different color shirts.

The fifth person has different hairstyles, different facial expressions, and different color shirts.

CHAPTER 6

MULTITASKING

Exercise 1 (page 84)

Name the baby version of each animal

1. Cat: kitten
2. Goat: kid
3. Pig: piglet
4. Horse: foal
5. Dog: puppy
6. Bird: chick
7. Kangaroo: joey
8. Sheep: lamb
9. Goose: gosling

Exercise 2 (page 85)

Name the continent for each country

1. India: Asia
2. Canada: North America
3. Indonesia: Asia
4. Angola: Africa
5. France: Europe
6. Brazil: South America
7. Madagascar: Africa
8. Algeria: Africa
9. Iran: Asia

Exercise 3 (page 86)
Name the fairy tale

1. Jack and Jill
2. Little Red Riding Hood
3. Hansel and Gretel
4. The Tortoise and the Hare
5. Three Little Pigs
6. Cinderella
7. Snow White and the Seven Dwarves
8. Rumpelstiltskin
9. The Princess and the Pea (alternate answer: Frog)

Exercise 4 (page 87)
Examples of dishes containing

1. Cinnamon: Hot apple cider
2. Jalapeños: Jalapeño poppers
3. Flour: Pancakes
4. Cream: Chocolate mousse
5. Maple syrup: Maple-roasted bacon
6. Onions: Meatloaf
7. Marshmallows: S'mores
8. Black olives: Enchiladas
9. Spinach: Eggs florentine

MENTAL COMPARISONS
Exercise 1 (page 88)
Peppers

1. Habanero: 350,000 SHU
2. Devil's Tongue: 300,000 SHU
3. Carolina Cayenne: 125,000 SHU
4. Tabasco: 50,000 SHU
5. Serrano: 23,000 SHU
6. Jalapeño: 10,000 SHU
7. Chipotle: 8,000 SHU
8. Poblano: 2,000 SHU
9. Pepperoncini: 900 SHU
10. Bell pepper: 0 SHU

Exercise 2 (page 88)
Shark lengths

1. Great white shark (25 feet)
2. Thresher shark (18 feet)
3. Great blue shark (15 feet)
4. Hammerhead shark (14 feet)
5. Nurse shark (13 feet)
6. Oceanic whitetip shark (11feet)
7. Whitetip shark (7 feet)
8. Blacktip shark (6 feet)

Exercise 3 (page 89)

State sizes

1.	Alaska	570,641 square miles
2.	Texas	261,914 square miles
3.	California	155,973 square miles
4.	Montana	145,556 square miles
5.	New Mexico	121,365 square miles
6.	Arizona	113,642 square miles
7.	Nevada	109,806 square miles
8.	Oregon	96,003 square miles
9.	Utah	82,168 square miles
10.	Minnesota	79,617 square miles
11.	Michigan	56,539 square miles

Exercise 4 (page 90)

Planets

1. Mercury: 1,516 miles (2,440 kilometers) radius; about a third the size of Earth

2. Mars: 2,106 miles (3,390 kilometers) radius; about half the size of Earth

3. Venus: 3,760 miles (6,052 kilometers) radius; only slightly smaller than Earth

4. Earth: 3,959 miles (6,371 kilometers) radius

5. Neptune: 15,299 miles (24,622 kilometers) radius; only slightly smaller than Uranus

6. Uranus: 15,759 miles (25,362 kilometers) radius; four times larger than Earth

7. Saturn: 36,184 miles (58,232 kilometers) radius; nine times larger than Earth

8. Jupiter: 43,441 miles (69,911 kilometers) radius; 11 times larger than Earth

Exercise 5 (page 91)
Sports

1. Soccer: 3.5 billion
2. Cricket: 2.5 billion
3. Basketball: 2.2 billion
4. Field hockey: 2 billion
5. Tennis: 1 billion

6. Volleyball: 900 million
7. Table tennis: 850 million
8. Baseball: 500 million
9. American football: 410 million and Rugby: 410 million (tied)

CHAPTER 7

THINK FAST

Exercises 1–5 (pages 95–97): Alphabet suggested/possible answers:

	Colors	Food	City	Plant	Use with Hands
A	amber	apple	Arcata	acacia	axe
B	blue	burger	Boston	bamboo	bat
C	charcoal	carp	Charleston	cactus	can opener
D	dark green	donut	Denver	daffodil	dart
E	eggplant	eggs	Eureka	eucalyptus	earplugs
F	fuchsia	falafel	Fairfax	fern	fan
G	gold	grains	Gainesville	gardenia	gloves
H	hazel	honey	Harrisburg	hawthorn	hammer
I	ivory	ice cream	Indianapolis	iris	ice pick

CONTINUED

	Colors	Food	City	Plant	Use with Hands
J	jade	jelly	Jacksonville	jasmine	jar
K	khaki	kebabs	Kansas City	kale	kite
L	lavender	lemons	Louisville	lotus	latch
M	maroon	milk	Memphis	magnolia	matches
N	navy blue	naan	Nashville	nettle	napkin
O	ochre	olives	Okinawa	oak	oven knob
P	periwinkle	pears	Portland	palm	pliers
Q	quartz	quiche	Québec City	Queen Anne's lace	quill
R	red	ramen	Rangpur	ranunculus	radio
S	saffron	spaghetti	San Francisco	seaweed	saw
T	teal	tiramisu	Toronto	thistle	tablet
U	ultramarine	upside-down cake	Ulm	umbrella pine	ukulele
V	violet	vanilla beans	Venice	violet	valve
W	white	watermelon	Wellington	walnut	wagon
X	xanthic	xylitol (common sweetener)	Xalapa	xeranthemum	xylophone
Y	yellow	yogurt	York	yew	yo-yo
Z	zucchini green	zucchini	Zabol	zucchini	zipper

Exercise 1 (page 98)

Time Tracker

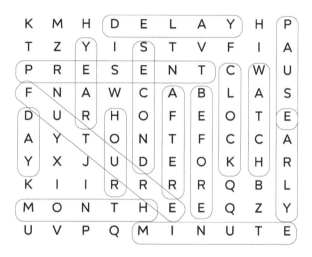

Exercise 2 (page 99)

Birding

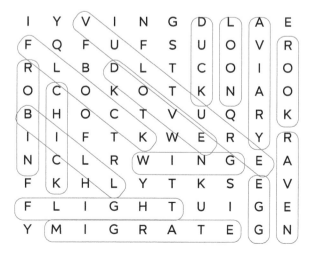

Exercise 3 (page 100)

Ahoy, sailor!

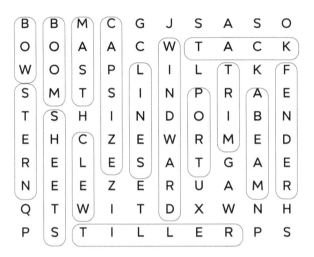

Exercise 4 (page 101)

Herbs and Spices

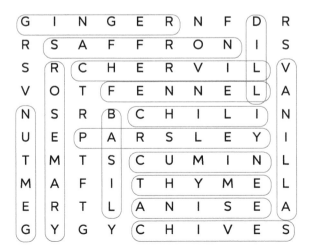

Exercise 5 (page 102)

Weather

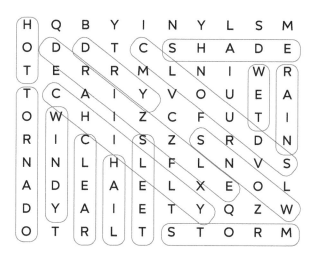

Exercise 6 (page 103)

Flowers

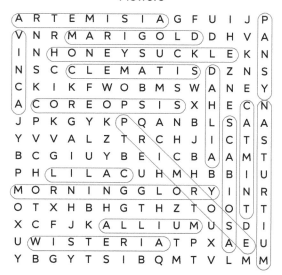

THE ODD ONES OUT

Exercises 1–4 (pages 104–105)

Sports

1. Track
2. Boxing
3. Ultimate Frisbee
4. Competitive swimming
5. Rowing
6. Wiffle ball
7. Roller derby
8. Crew
9. Pool
10. Weightlifting
11. Golf
12. Surfing
13. Cricket
14. Snowboarding
15. Cheerleading
16. Football
17. Rugby
18. Baseball
19. Skateboarding
20. Tennis

European countries

1. Jersey
2. Faroe Islands
3. Monaco
4. Vatican City
5. Isle of Man
6. Malta
7. Estonia
8. Slovenia
9. Switzerland
10. Bulgaria
11. Belarus
12. Sweden
13. Liechtenstein
14. Albania
15. Portugal
16. Iceland
17. Belgium
18. Spain
19. Germany
20. Finland

Animals

1. Bumblebee
2. Musk deer
3. Elk
4. Beaver
5. Hog
6. Cricket
7. Giraffe
8. Mink
9. Eagle owl
10. Lovebird
11. Dung beetle
12. Thorny devil
13. Bull
14. Wildcat
15. Whale
16. Pig
17. Shrew
18. Hare
19. Quail
20. Jaguar

Household items

1. Pencil
2. Bag
3. Bookmark
4. Waste bin
5. Eyeliner
6. Lampshade
7. Guitar
8. Rug
9. Outlet
10. Water bottle
11. Monitor
12. USB drive
13. Leg warmers
14. Speakers
15. Slipper
16. Bottle cap
17. Mirror
18. Sofa
19. Plastic fork
20. Magnet

Strategy Check (page 106)

"cheers to your health, wealth, and wisdom!"

GLOSSARY

association: Linking pieces of information together to strengthen future recall.

chunking: Grouping pieces of information together to form more manageable "chunks," which makes for fewer overall pieces to remember but with greater overall information recall.

cue: A reminder of information to be recalled; cues can be visual, auditory, tactile, or related to time.

elaboration: Similar to association, elaboration relies on already known information to create a greater meaning and stronger recall of learned information.

long-term memory: Information held for an extended period of time (typically longer than 30 minutes).

procedural memory: A subtype of implicit memory allowing us to carry out a sequence of actions based on prior experience/practice; it is often unconscious.

rehearsal: Repeating information over and over in order to keep it active in our minds or with the aim of committing it to long-term memory.

short-term memory: Sometimes called primary memory, short-term memory is the active retention of information in our minds before it goes to processing in the brain (but not yet working with it, which would then make it working memory).

RESOURCES

APPS

Brainscape: Brainscape.com, a responsive flash-card app based on spaced repetition

Eidetic: EideticApp.com, spaced repetition tool for information across various types and categories

Elevate: ElevateApp.com, a brain training tool designed to build communication and analytical skills

WEBSITES

BrainFacts: BrainFacts.org, interactive exploratory tool for examining the brain, its structures and functions, and various abilities and diseases.

Harvard Health Publishing: Health.Harvard.edu/topics/improving-memory, includes tips to improve concentration.

Mouse Party: Learn.Genetics.Utah.edu/content/addiction/mouse, traces the effects of recreational substances on the brain through a novel interactive cartoon interface.

Sleep Foundation: SleepFoundation.org, resource for common sleep disorders.

BOOKS

Atomic Habits: An Easy & Proven Way to Build Good Habits & Break Bad Ones by James Clear, a guide to better living, including a framework for habit formation to apply to everyday habits.

The Great Mental Models: General Thinking Concepts by Rhiannon Beaubien and Shane Parrish, a conceptual guide from the curators of "ideas and mental models that history's brightest minds have used to live lives of purpose."

Mindset: The New Psychology of Success by Carol Dweck, insight into the dramatic influence of how we think about our talents and abilities.

Moonwalking with Einstein: The Art and Science of Remembering Everything by Joshua Foer, a story of the journey toward competing in memory competitions.

REFERENCES

Asok, A., F. Leroy, J. B. Raymon, and E. R. Kandel. "Molecular Mechanisms of the Memory Trace." *Trends in Neurosciences* 42, no. 1 (January 2019): 14–22. doi:doi.org/10.1016/j.tins.2018.10.005.

Boyd, Robynne. "Do People Only Use 10 Percent of Their Brains?" Scientific American. Scientific American, February 7, 2008. ScientificAmerican.com /article/do-people-only-use-10-percent-of-their-brains.

Cowan, Nelson. "The Magical Number 4 in Short-term Memory: A Reconsid eration of Mental Storage Capacity." *Behavioral and Brain Sciences* 24, no. 1 (February 2001): 87–114. Cambridge.org/core/journals/behavioral-and -brain-sciences/article/magical-number-4-in-shortterm-memory-a -reconsideration-of-mental-storage-capacity/44023F1147D4A1D44 BDC0AD226838496.

Csikszentmihalyi, Mihaly. *Flow: The Psychology of Optimal Experience.* New York, NY: Harper Collins Publishers, 1991.

Dalai Lama Center for Peace and Education. "Dan Siegel – 'Flipping Your Lid:' A Scientific Explanation." YouTube Video, 7:27. February 28, 2012. https://youtu.be/G0T_2NNoC68.

Demaree, David. "Google and Cognitive Overhead." Accessed March 8, 2021. Demaree.space/google-and-cognitive-overhead.

Lezak, Muriel Deutsch., Diane B. Howieson, Erin D. Bigler, and Daniel Tranel. *Neuropsychological Assessment.* 5th ed. Oxford: Oxford University Press, 2004.

Miller, Earl K., Mikael Lundqvist, and André M. Bastos. "Working Memory 2.0." *Neuron* 100, no. 2 (October 2018): 463–75. doi:10.1016/j.neuron.2018.09.023.

Moran, Rani, Michael Zehetleitner, Heinrich René Liesefeld, Hermann J. Müller, and Marius Usher. "Serial vs. Parallel Models of Attention in Visual Search: Accounting for Benchmark RT-distributions." *Psychonomic Bulletin & Review* 23, no. 5 (2015): 1300–315. doi:10.3758/s13423-015-0978-1.

Parrish, Shane, and Rhiannon Beaubien. *The Great Mental Models: General Thinking Concepts.* 1. Vol. 1. Ottawa, Canada: Latticework Publishing Inc., 2019.

Parsons, Michael W., Thomas A. Hammeke, and P. J. Snyder. *Clinical Neuro psychology: A Pocket Handbook for Assessment.* Washington, DC: Ameri can Psychological Association, 2014.

Rose, Nathan S., S. Hale, H. L. Roediger, III, and J. Meyerson. "Similarities and Differences between Working Memory and Long-Term Memory: Evidence from the Levels-of-Processing Span Task." *Journal of Experimental Psychology: Learning, Memory, and Cognition* 36, no. 2 (March 2010): 471. doi:10.1037/a0018405.

"Top 10 Most Popular Sports in The World." Sports Show, March 23, 2021. SportsShow.net/top-10-most-popular-sports-in-the-world.

Unsworth, N., and R. W. Engle. "The Nature of Individual Differences in Working Memory Capacity: Active Maintenance in Primary Memory and Controlled Search from Secondary Memory." *Psychology Review* 114, no. 1 (January 2007): 104. doi:10.1037/0033-295X.114.1.104.

Waldum, Emily R., Carolyn L. Dufault, and Mark A. McDaniel. "Prospective Memory Training." *Journal of Applied Gerontology* 35, no. 11 (September 2016): 1211–234. doi:10.1177/0733464814559418.

ABOUT THE AUTHOR

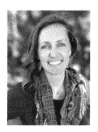 **Alexis Olson, PhD,** specializes in neuropsychological evaluations and therapy for individuals affected by brain injury, chronic pain/illness, and caregiving. She regularly provides cognitive training, involving learning and practicing compensatory cognitive strategies in everyday life situations. Her background includes a PhD in clinical psychology from the University of California, Santa Barbara. Find out more about Dr. Alexis Olson at DoctorOlson.com.